Claudia Westermann

Blutübertragbare Virushepatitis C bei Beschäftigten im Gesundheitswesen

Claudia Westermann

Blutübertragbare Virushepatitis C bei Beschäftigten im Gesundheitswesen

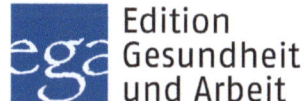
Edition
Gesundheit
und Arbeit

© 2019
Edition Gesundheit und Arbeit,
Schriftenreihe des CVcare, Band 12
Blutübertragbare Virushepatitis C bei Beschäftigten
im Gesundheitswesen

Universitätsklinikum Hamburg-Eppendorf (UKE),
CVcare | Bethanien-Höfe Eppendorf
Martinistraße 52, 20246 Hamburg
www.uke.de

Herausgeber
Prof. Dr. med. Albert Nienhaus
a.nienhaus@uke.de

Autorin
Claudia Westermann

Redaktion
Elisabeth Muth

Gestaltung
Ethel Knop

Verlag
tredition GmbH, Halenreie 40-44, 22359 Hamburg
ISBN: 978-3-7482-8319-5

Bibliografische Information der Deutschen Nationalbibliothek
Die Deutsche Nationalbibliothek verzeichnet diese Publikation in der Deutschen Nationalbibliografie; detaillierte bibliografische Daten sind im Internet über http://dnb.d-nb.de abrufbar.

Inhaltsverzeichnis

Vorwort Herausgeber

Die Edition Gesundheit und Arbeit (ega) ist eine Schriftenreihe des Competenz-zentrums für Epidemiologie und Versorgungsforschung bei Pflegeberufen (CVcare) am Universitätsklinikum Hamburg-Eppendorf (UKE).

Mit der *ega* soll die Diskussion im deutschsprachigen Raum über effektive und effi-ziente Wege zur Verbesserung des Gesundheitsschutzes, der betrieblichen Gesund-heitsförderung sowie des betrieblichen Gesundheitsmanagements unter besonderer Berücksichtigung der betrieblichen Wiedereingliederung sowie der Rehabilitation ge-fördert werden. Die *ega* ist eine Plattform für interdisziplinäre Beiträge aus der arbeitsweltbezogenen Gesundheitsforschung. Die Disziplinen Psychologie, Arbeits-medizin, Gesundheitswissenschaften, Gesundheitsökonomie, Rehabilitations- und Ver-sorgungsforschung sollen damit näher zusammengeführt und zum gegenseitigen Austausch angeregt werden.

Das CVcare ist Teil des Institutes für Versorgungsforschung in der Dermatologie und bei Pflegeberufen (IVDP) am UKE. Die Grundfinanzierung des CVcare wird durch eine Stiftung der Berufsgenossenschaft für Gesundheitsdienst und Wohlfahrtspflege (BGW) sichergestellt. Das CVcare kooperiert daher eng mit der BGW und hier insbesondere mit deren Forschungsbereich Grundlagen der Prävention und Rehabilitation (GPR).

Das CVcare stellt epidemiologische Daten zur Arbeits- und Gesundheitssituation von Pflegekräften und anderen Beschäftigten im Gesundheitswesen und in der Wohlfahrtspflege zur Verfügung. Angebote zur arbeitsweltbezogenen Gesund-heitsförderung, Prävention und Rehabilitation werden unter besonderer Berück-sichtigung des demografischen Wandels im Sinne der Versorgungsforschung über-prüft. In praxisorientierten Projekten werden Vorschläge zur weiteren Verbesserung dieser Angebote entwickelt.

Schwerpunktthemen des CVcare sind die Arbeitssituation älterer Beschäftigter in der Pflege, arbeitsbedingte Beschwerden des Bewegungsapparates (MSB), Infektionsrisiken mit den Schwerpunkten Nadelstichverletzungen, Tuberkulose und multiresistente Erreger (MRE), psychosoziale Belastungen am Arbeitsplatz mit dem besonderen Schwerpunkt Gewalt am Arbeitsplatz sowie die Evaluation der Rehabilitationsleistungen der BGW und anderer Träger der gesetzlichen Unfall-versicherung (GUV).

Der zwölfte Band der Edition gibt die Promotionsarbeit „Blutübertragbare Virus-hepatitis C bei Beschäftigten im Gesundheitswesen" von Claudia Westermann wieder. Eine Hepatitis-C-Virus (HCV)-Infektion kann chronisch verlaufen und schwerwiegende Folgen für die Betroffenen haben: Leberzirrhose und Hepatozelluläres Karzinom. Die Zusammenhangsbegutachtung einer HCV-Infektion im Berufskrankheitenverfahren kann Probleme bereiten, da Nadelstichverletzungen als häufigste Ursache für eine beruflich bedingte Übertragung oftmals nicht erfasst oder gemeldet werden. Das systematische Review und die Metaanalyse zum beruflichen Infektionsrisiko von Claudia Westermann belegen ein erhöhtes Infektionsrisiko für ärztliches Personal, für Labormitarbeiter und für Beschäftigte mit Tätigkeiten, die zu Blutkontakten führen. Es gibt aber auch zwei sehr positive Entwicklungen bei der HCV-Infektion. Die Anzahl der Neuinfektionen bei Beschäftigten hat sich deutlich reduziert, wie Claudia Westermann in ihrer Analyse der BK-DOC-Daten der BGW zeigt. Für die mehr als 1.000 Versicherten mit einer bereits bestehenden beruflichen HCV-Infektion gibt es aber auch eine gute Nachricht. Seit dem Jahr 2014 stehen in Deutschland die sogenannten „Direct Acting Antivirals (DAA)" zur Verfügung, mit denen die Eliminierung der Viren auch bei schon lange bestehender Infektion fast immer gelingt. Selbst bei Versicherten mit einer Leberzirrhose gelang bei über 90 % die Eliminierung der Viren, wie Claudia Westermann in ihrer dritten Arbeit zur Analyse der DAA-Behandlungen bei Versicherten mit einer HCV bedingten Berufskrankheit zeigt.

Ich hatte die Freude, die Promotionsarbeit von Claudia Westermann zusammen mit Prof. Dr. Monika Bullinger, Institut für medizinische Psychologie, und Prof. Dr. Ralf Reintjes, Hochschule für angewandte Wissenschaften (HAW), Hamburg, zu betreuen. Für die Unterstützung und gute Zusammenarbeit möchte ich mich hier bei beiden bedanken.

Es freut mich, dem interessierten Leser die Arbeit zur Hepatitis C bei Beschäftigten im Gesundheitswesen in der Schriftenreihe *ega* zur Verfügung stellen zu können.

Hamburg, im Mai 2019   Prof. Dr. med. Albert Nienhaus

Zusammenfassung

Einleitung

Infektionen mit Hepatitis-C-Viren (HCV) gehören zu den häufigsten Infektions-krankheiten weltweit. Sie verursachen potenziell schwere Krankheitsverläufe, die zu Berufsunfähigkeit und zum Tod führen können. Hierbei entstehen erhebliche Kosten. Die Übertragung des Hepatitis-C-Virus erfolgt von Mensch zu Mensch, eine Schutzimpfung gibt es bislang nicht. Beschäftigte im Gesundheitswesen (BiG) haben aufgrund ihrer beruflichen Tätigkeiten Kontakt zu infizierten Patienten. Die beruflich verursachte HCV-Infektion ist Inhalt dieser Arbeit. In der ersten Studie wird der Ursachenzusammenhang zwischen beruflicher Tätigkeit und einer Infektion mit HCV bei BiG untersucht. In den zwei weiteren Studien werden die assoziierten Kosten der HCV als Berufskrankheit (BK) sowie die Behandlungserfolge der neuen direkt antiviralen Therapien (direct-acting antiviral agents, DAA) bei den Beschäftigten analysiert.

Methoden

Die Frage der beruflichen Exposition der BiG im Vergleich zu Kontrollen wurde anhand einer Metaanalyse zur HCV-Prävalenz in Studie 1 untersucht. Es wurden berufsspezifische Effektschätzer ermittelt. Die zweite und die dritte Studie analy-sieren anhand von Routinedaten einer Unfallversicherung die Kosten der HCV als BK sowie die Ergebnisse DAA-basierter Therapien bei BiG. Anhand einer multiva-riaten Regressionsanalyse wurden Prädiktoren für den Behandlungserfolg zwölf Wochen nach Therapieende (SVR12) ermittelt.

Ergebnisse

Die gepoolte Analyse ergab ein statistisch signifikant erhöhtes OR für eine HCV-Infektion bei BiG im Vergleich zur Allgemeinbevölkerung (OR 1,6; 95%-CI 1,03-2,42). Die Analyse für Berufsgruppen zeigte im Vergleich zu Kontrollen ein erhöhtes OR für eine HCV-Infektion bei Ärzten (OR 2,7), Labormitarbeitern (OR 2,20) und bei BiG, die ein hohes Risiko für Blutkontakte aufgrund invasiver Tätigkeiten haben (OR 2,7). Für die HCV-Infektion als BK ist ein anhaltend rückläufiger Trend bei der Anzahl der Fälle zu beobachten bei gleichzeitig steigenden Kosten. Die Kosten wurden überwiegend von den steigenden Ausgaben für Rentenleistungen und seit 2012 für medikamentöse Therapien bestimmt. Im untersuchten Kollektiv erreichten HCV-Infizierte hohe SVR12-Raten (94 %) durch die eingesetzten DAA-Therapien. Als Prädiktor für einen statistisch signifikant verminderten Therapieerfolg erwies sich eine Zirrhose (86 % SVR12, p=0,006).

Fazit

Durch die antiviralen Medikamente haben BiG mit einer HCV-Infektion neben einer verbesserten gesundheitlichen auch eine günstigere berufliche Prognose. Angesichts der hohen Erfolgsraten der DAA-Therapien werden zukünftig progrediente Verläufe mit Leberschädigungen und deren Folgen vermieden. Arbeitsmedizinische Maßnahmen wie der Schutz vor Nadelstichverletzungen zählen weiterhin zu den wichtigsten Präventionsstrategien zur Vermeidung von (Re)-Infektionen mit HCV.

Abstract

Introduction

Infections with viral hepatitis C (HCV) are among the most common infectious diseases worldwide. They cause potentially severe disease progressions that can lead to disability and death. This results in considerable costs. The hepatitis C virus is transmitted from person to person, and no vaccination is available to date. Healthcare workers (HCWs) have contact with infected patients as a result of their professional activities. The occupationally acquired HCV infection is the content of this piece of work. The first study investigates the causal relationship between occupational activity and HCV infection in HCWs. In the two other studies the associated costs of HCV as an occupational disease and the success of the new direct-acting antiviral agents (DAA) in treating employees are analysed.

Methods

The question of occupational exposure of HCWs in comparison to controls was investigated using a meta-analysis of HCV prevalence in Study 1, occupational effect estimators were determined. The second and third study analysed the costs of HCV as an occupational disease and the results of DAA-based therapies in HCWs on the basis of routine data from accident insurance. Using a multivariate regression analysis predictors for treatment success were determined twelve weeks after the end of treatment (SVR12).

Results

The pooled analysis revealed a statistically significantly elevated OR for HCV infection in HCWs compared to the general population (OR 1.6; 95% CI 1.03-2.42). The analysis for occupational groups showed an increased OR compared to controls for HCV infection for physicians (OR 2.7), laboratory staff (OR 2.20) and for HCWs who have a high risk of blood contact due to invasive activities (OR 2.7). For HCV infection as an occupational disease, a continuing downward trend in the number of cases can be observed with simultaneously rising costs. The costs were mainly determined by the rising expenses for pension benefits and, since 2012, for drug therapies. In the investigated collective, HCV-infected persons achieved high SVR12 rates (94%) through the DAA therapies used.

Existing cirrhosis proved to be a predictor for statistically significantly reduced treatment success (86 % SVR12, p=0,006).

Conclusion

Thanks to antiviral drugs, HCWs with an HCV infection not only have an improved health but also a more favourable occupational prognosis. The high success rates of DAA therapies will in future prevent progressive courses with liver damage and its consequences. Occupational medical measures such as protection against needlestick injuries continue to be among the most important preventive measures against (re)infection with HCV.

Publikationsliste

Westermann C, Peters C, Lisiak B, Lamberti M, Nienhaus A.
The prevalence of hepatitis C among healthcare workers: a systematic review and meta-analysis
Occupational and environmental medicine 2015;72(12):880-8

Westermann C, Dulon M, Wendeler D, Nienhaus A.
Hepatitis C among healthcare personnel: secondary data analyses of costs and trends for hepatitis C infections with occupational causes
Journal of Occupational Medicine and Toxicology 2016;11:52

Westermann C, Wendeler D, Nienhaus A.
Hepatitis C in healthcare personnel: secondary data analysis of therapies with direct-acting antiviral agents
Journal of Occupational Medicine and Toxicology 2018;13:16

Die deutsche Übersetzung der ersten beiden Studien wurde in Buchbeiträgen des Ecomed Verlags veröffentlicht:

RiRe – Risiken und Ressourcen in Gesundheitsdienst und Wohlfahrtspflege Band 2 (2015)
S. 285–320 und **Band 3 (2018)** S. 97–114, Nienhaus, A. (Hrsg.),
ecomed: Landsberg am Lech

Eine Zusammenfassung der zweiten Studie wurde in einer deutschen Fachzeitschrift veröffentlicht:

Hepatitis-C-Infektionen bei Beschäftigten im Gesundheitswesen. Eine Zusammenfassung von Trends und Kosten

Westermann C, Dulon M, Wendeler D, Nienhaus A.
Arbeitsmedizin, Sozialmedizin, Umweltmedizin 2017;52: 41-42

1 Synopse

1.1   Einleitung

Virale Hepatitiden sind weltweit verbreitet und zählen zu den häufigsten blut-übertragbaren Infektionskrankheiten. Gemäß aktuellen Schätzungen der Welt-gesundheitsorganisation (WHO) starben im Jahr 2015 weltweit circa 1,34 Millionen Menschen an den Folgen einer chronischen viralen Hepatitis (Typ B oder C). Die Mortalitätsrate entspricht der für Tuberkulose (TBC) beziehungsweise übersteigt die für das humane Immundefizienz-Virus (HIV). Im Gegensatz zu TBC und HIV, die seit Jahren eine kontinuierliche Abnahme bei der Sterberate verzeichnen, steigt diese bei den viralen Hepatitisinfektionen (B/C) weiterhin an (1). Die chronischen Hepatitis-B-Virus(HBV)- und Hepatitis-C-Virus(HCV)-Infektionen zählen zu den bedeutendsten Ursachen von Leberzirrhose und des Leberzellkarzinoms (2, 3). Die akute HCV-Infektion bleibt häufig unbemerkt und geht mit einer hohen Chronizität einher. Die chronische Hepatitis C (CHC) ist mit Morbidität und Mortalität assoziiert und zeichnet sich als ein weltweites Public-Health-Problem ab (1). Nach Angaben der WHO sind circa 71 Millionen Menschen an einer CHC erkrankt, wobei der größte Anteil der Betroffenen keine Kenntnis davon hat (1). Die zunehmende globale Anzahl Infizierter stellt eine Gefährdung für Beschäftigte im Gesundheitswesen (BiG) dar (4, 5). Sie haben durch verletzungsträchtige Tätigkeiten ein hohes Risiko für eine HCV-Infektion (6, 7). Der Zusammenhang zwischen beruflicher Tätigkeit und einer HCV-Infektion ist für die Unfallversicherungsträger (UV-Träger) eine zentrale Frage im Berufskrankheiten(BK)-Feststellungsverfahren. Der Ursachenzusammenhang zwischen Einwirkung und Erkrankung muss wahrscheinlich sein. Die ursächliche Einwirkung ist aufgrund des inapparenten und häufig unspezifischen Verlaufs der HCV-Infektion zeitlich kaum zu ermitteln. Verletzungen des medizinischen Personals sind an der Tagesordnung (7). Würde ein Vollbeweis der HCV-Übertragung mit Angaben zur Indexperson, zum Zeitpunkt und zum Übertragungsmodus not-wendig sein, würden die meisten beruflich erworbenen HCV-Infektionskrankheiten nicht anerkannt (8). Deshalb reicht es zu belegen, dass Tätigkeiten ausgeführt wur-den, die mit einem erhöhten Infektionsrisiko verbunden sind. Um die gesetzlichen Voraussetzungen für eine BK zu prüfen, sind Regelungen erforderlich, die durch evidenzbasierte Daten gestützt werden. Aufgrund der inkonsistenten Studienlage ist es für die BiG schwierig gewesen zu belegen, dass die HCV-Infektion durch eine beruflich bedingte Exposition erworben wurde.

Die hier vorgelegte kumulative Dissertation ist aus dieser Anforderung und der gesetzlichen Pflicht der UV-Träger heraus entstanden, sich an Forschungsvorhaben zur Weiterentwicklung des BK-Rechts zu beteiligen und diese zu fördern (§ 9 Abs. 8 SGB VII (9)). Die zunächst dargestellte Metaanalyse schafft eine wichtige Voraussetzung zur Beantwortung der Frage nach dem beruflichen Ursachenzusammenhang. Noch vor wenigen Jahren ging die Diagnose einer HCV-Infektion für BiG mit einer gesundheitlich und beruflich schlechten Prognose einher. Lange Zeit galt die CHC als schwer therapierbar, neuropsychiatrische Symptome der chronischen Infektion wurden potenziell durch Interferon-alpha-Behandlungen verstärkt (10). Im Weiteren beschäftigt sich diese Dissertation mit den Kosten und Trends der berufsbedingten CHC. Seit der Entwicklung von neuen, direkt antiviral wirksamen Medikamenten (direct–acting antiviral agents, DAA) zeichnet sich eine Trendwende bei der Behandlung der HCV-Infektion ab. Die Ergebnisse der DAA-Therapien bei BiG und deren potenziellen Auswirkungen auf die BK-Folgen sind Inhalt der dritten Publikation.

1.2 Hintergrund

Das HCV wurde Ende der 1980er Jahre isoliert und als hauptursächlich für die bis dahin als Non-A-non-B-Hepatitis bezeichnete Infektion identifiziert (11). Erst im Jahr 1989 wurden die ersten Tests zum Nachweis einer HCV-Infektion möglich (12, 13). Das HCV gehört zu den Flaviviren (Flaviviridae). Es ist ein umhülltes Einzelstrang-Ribonukleinsäure-(RNA)-Virus mit positiver Polarität. Das HCV-Genom besteht aus strukturellen Hüllproteinen (E1, E2, p7), einem strukturellen Kernprotein (Core) und aus nicht strukturellen (NS)-Proteinen (NS2, NS3, NS4A, NS4B, NS5A, NS5B) (14–16). Die Genomreplikation erfolgt ausschließlich im Zytoplasma der Wirtzelle. Als natürliche Wirtzellen gelten menschliche Leberepithelzellen (Hepatozyten). Für die intrazelluläre Replikation sind die NS-Proteine verantwortlich; für diesen Vorgang werden virale Enzyme, die sogenannten Proteasen, benötigt. Die DAA basieren auf der Grundlage der Entschlüsselung des HCV-Genoms und seines Replikationszyklus. Sie wirken als Inhibitoren (Substanzen, die chemische Vorgänge einschränken bzw. verhindern) und werden im Zyklus der viralen Replikation eingesetzt. Als spezifische Enzyminhibitoren unterbinden DAA unter anderem die effiziente NS2-NS3-Spaltung, die als zwingende Voraussetzung für den erfolgreichen Zusammenbau der viralen Replikationskomplexe (NS5A-Hyperphosphorylierung als Ausdruck erfolgreichen Viruszusammenbaus) gilt (17).

Hohe Replikationsraten, verbunden mit Fehlern in der viralen Polymerase, sind verantwortlich für die ausgeprägte Variabilität des Hepatitis-C-Virus (15). Aktuell sind sieben große Genotypen (GT, arabische Ziffern 1–7) und zahlreiche Subtypen (kleine Buchstaben) bekannt (18). Weltweit am häufigsten verbreitet ist der GT 1 (46 %) in Europa mit Subtyp b, in Nordamerika, Großbritannien, Skandinavien und Australien mit Subtyp a. HCV ist eine blutübertragbare Infektion, sie bleibt aufgrund ihres inapparenten Verlaufs häufig unbemerkt. In bis zu 85 % der Fälle nimmt die Infektion einen chronischen Verlauf, nicht selten bleibt sie undiagnostiziert bis zum Auftreten von Leberschädigungen oder anderen Krankheitsfolgen (1, 19). Bei ausbleibender adäquater Behandlung führt eine Entzündung der Leber langfristig zur Schädigung des Organgewebes. Verantwortlich dafür ist hauptsächlich die Immunantwort auf die virusinfizierten Zellen. Allerdings gibt es Hinweise darauf, dass das Virus selbst seine Wirtzelle schädigt (14, 15). Die CHC ist mit einer hohen Morbiditätsrate und mit einer Minderung der gesundheitsbezogenen Lebensqualität assoziiert. Betroffene leiden unter anderem an Müdigkeit, Abgeschlagenheit, Einschränkung der Leistungsfähigkeit und subklinischen kognitiven Störungen. Es besteht ferner ein größeres Risiko für die Entwicklung einer Leberzirrhose und eines Leberzellkarzinoms (19). Die CHC ist die Hauptindikation für eine Lebertransplantation (63 %) in Europa (2). Darüber hinaus können vielfältige extrahepatische Manifestationen auftreten. Als gesichert gelten unter anderem assoziierte depressive Symptome, Diabetes mellitus und maligne lymphoproliferative Erkrankungen. Mehrere Studien weisen zudem auf Beeinträchtigungen bestimmter zentralnervöser Funktionen und der Neurotransmission hin (20). Bislang gibt es für die Hepatitis C keine Schutzimpfung.

Diagnostik

Die Diagnostik bei Verdacht auf eine HCV-Infektion besteht aus einem Nachweis spezifischer Antikörper gegen HCV (mittels Immunoassay, z. B. Anti-HCV-EIA) und aus einem Nachweis von Virus-Ribonukleinsäure (RNA) (z. B. durch polymerase chain reaction, PCR, oder Nukleinsäure-Amplifikationstechnologie, NAT). Der alleinige Nachweis von HCV-Antikörpern erlaubt keine Unterscheidung zwischen einer ausgeheilten und einer aktiven HCV-Erkrankung. Um den Anteil der aktiven HCV-Infektionen (akute und chronische) zu erfassen, muss ein direkter Erregernachweis erfolgen (HCV-RNA). Als akut wird die Infektion in den ersten sechs Monaten definiert, wobei diese labortechnisch selten zu diagnostizieren ist. Vor der Serokonversion sind bei einem positiven HCV-RNA-Nachweis die HCV-Antikörper noch nicht nachweisbar. Das serodiagnostische Fenster beträgt sieben bis acht

Wochen. HCV-RNA ist bereits ein bis zwei Wochen nach einer Infektion nachweisbar. Eine Infektion, die länger als sechs Monate besteht, wird als CHC-Infektion bezeichnet (19).

Epidemiologie

Die HCV-Infektion ist global verbreitet. Nach aktuellen Schätzungen der WHO haben circa 71 Millionen Menschen eine CHC, das entspricht etwa 1% der Weltbevölkerung (1). Die höchste CHC-Prävalenz wird für die östliche Mittelmeerregion (2,3%) geschätzt, gefolgt von Europa (1,5%). Für die anderen WHO-Regionen liegt die Prävalenzschätzung zwischen 0,5 und 1% (1).

Die WHO schätzt die Zahl der CHC-infizierten Menschen in Europa auf circa 14 Millionen, hervorgerufen zu einem großen Anteil durch injizierende Drogenkonsumenten. Die Inzidenz und Prävalenz der HCV-Infektion variiert zwischen den Ländern. Die Anti-HCV-Prävalenz beträgt in Belgien, Niederlanden und Irland 0,1%, in Italien 5,9% (21). Die Anti-HCV-Rate gibt Auskunft über eine erfolgte Immunantwort. Aktuelle Schätzungen der Anti-HCV-Prävalenz liegen aus der „Studie zur Gesundheit Erwachsener in Deutschland" (DEGS) vor, Deutschland zählt mit einer Prävalenz von 0,3% (95%-CI 0,1-0,5) zu den Niedrigprävalenzländern (22). Allerdings fehlen in dieser Studie Angaben zu Risikogruppen, wie z.B. injizierende (intravenös) Drogenkonsumierende (IVD), Personen aus Justizvollzugsanstalten und medizinisches Personal. In Deutschland besteht für HCV nach dem Infektionsschutzgesetz (§ 6 IfSG (23)) eine namentliche Meldepflicht für Ärzte und diagnostische Institutionen (Labore). Gemäß der Falldefinitionsanpassung aus dem Jahr 2015 fallen unter diese Meldepflicht nur aktive Fälle mit einem direkten Erregernachweis (Nachweis von HCV-RNA oder von HCV-Core-Antigen). Ein HCV-Antikörpernachweis ohne direkten Erregernachweis hat vor der Definitionsanpassung zur Meldung bereits ausgeheilter oder gemeldeter Fälle geführt. Daten des Robert Koch-Instituts zeigen, dass über einen Zeitraum von 17 Jahren die übermittelten Jahresinzidenzen von anfänglich 9.000 HCV-Erstdiagnosen seit 2005 kontinuierlich bis auf circa 5.500 im Jahr 2009 sanken und sich stabil auf diesem Niveau bis 2013 gehalten haben (*Abb.1*). Nach einem Anstieg im Jahr 2014 (mögliche Zunahme der diagnostischen Testung durch verbesserte Therapieoptionen) kam es bis einschließlich 2016 zu einem weiteren Rückgang. Zu erwähnen ist hierbei die zum 1.1.2015 in Kraft getretene Änderung der Falldefinition für HCV. Im Jahr 2017 kam es erneut zu einem leichten Anstieg, dieser ist vor allem auf eine Zunahme der Fallzahlen bei Männern zurückzuführen. Insgesamt weisen Frauen geringere Fallzahlen als Männer auf (24).

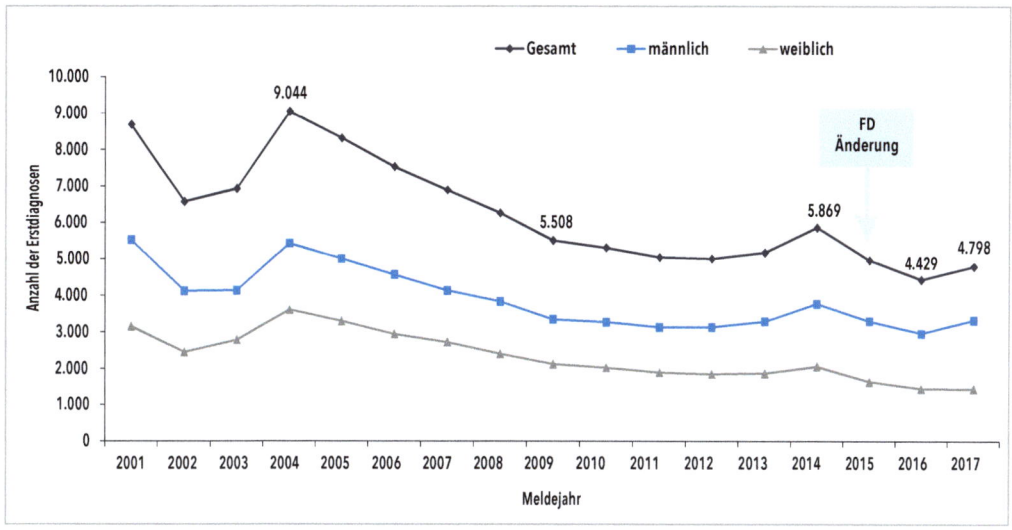

Abbildung 1 „Übermittelte Hepatitis-C-Erstdiagnosen gesamt und nach Geschlecht" (nur Fälle, die der Referenzdefinition entsprechen), Deutschland, 2001 bis 2017 (Datenstand 1. März 2018) (24)

Infektionsweg und Risikogruppen

Die Übertragung des HCV erfolgt von Mensch zu Mensch, hauptsächlich über Kontakt zu infektiösem Blut bei gleichzeitig bestehenden Verletzungen der Haut oder der Schleimhäute (25). Die HCV-RNA kann auch in anderen Körperflüssigkeiten nachweisbar sein (z. B. in Speichel, Tränen, Sperma, Muttermilch und Schweiß); eine Übertragung durch diese gilt als unwahrscheinlich (21). Zur Hauptrisikogruppe zählen injizierende (intravenös) Drogenkonsumierende (IVD) aufgrund des mehrfachen und gemeinsamen Verwendens von Injektionsutensilien. Nosokomiale Übertragungen stellen weltweit die Hauptursache für neue HCV-Infektionen dar, in Deutschland sind sie eher selten (26). Seit der Einführung der HCV-RNA-Testung für Blut und Blutpräparate im Jahr 1991 ist das Risiko einer Übertragung durch Blutprodukte in Deutschland und in anderen Industrieländern minimal. Eine sexuelle Übertragung ist durch ungeschützten verletzungsträchtigen Sex (Mann mit Mann, MSM) möglich, besonders betroffen sind HIV-positive Personen. Eine HIV-HCV-Koinfektion verläuft häufig mit einer starken Virämie, mit einem verminderten Behandlungserfolg und einer schnellen Progredienz zur Leberzirrhose (27). Es besteht ein vertikales Transmissionsrisiko, insbesondere während der Entbindung (28, 29).

Behandlung

Im Gegensatz zur HIV-Infektion kommt es bei 20 bis 30 % der HCV-Infizierten zu einer spontanen Viruseradikation (30). Ohne effektive Therapie beträgt der Median der CHC-Infektion bis zur Entwicklung einer Leberzirrhose 30 Jahre, 20 bis 30 % der Infizierten entwickeln bereits nach zehn bis zwanzig Jahren eine Leberzirrhose (31). Die Behandlung der HCV-Infektion basierte über Jahrzehnte auf Interferon-α, in der Regel als subkutane Injektionsgabe. Die Wirkung, vermittelt über Rezeptoren, beruht sowohl auf der Hemmung des Virusreplikationszyklus als auch auf einem immunmodulatorischen Effekt. Dieser wird über die Aktivierung der körpereigenen Killerzellen vermittelt. Eine adäquate T-Zell-Antwort wurde schon früh als entscheidender Faktor für die spontane Ausheilung der HCV-Infektion angenommen (32, 33). Darüber hinaus hat Interferon-α einen antitumoralen Effekt und wirkt direkt zytotoxisch. Diese Medikamenteneigenschaften führen zu zahlreichen systemischen, hämatologischen, psychischen, neurologischen, autoimmunen, gastrointestinalen und dermatologischen Nebenwirkungen, die häufig ausgeprägt verlaufen. Diese unerwünschten Ereignisse führten in der Vergangenheit gehäuft zu Dosisreduktionen und Therapieabbrüchen (33). Die Kombinationstherapie mit Ribavirin (RBV, synthetisch hergestelltes Nukleosid-Analogon) verbessert die Effektivität von Interferon-α im Vergleich zur Monotherapie (sustained virological response, SVR 38 bis 43 % statt 13 bis 19 %). Durch die Entwicklung von pegyliertem Interferon-α-2b (PEG-IFN) wurde die Halbwertszeit des Medikaments verlängert, sodass die Häufigkeit der Einnahme reduziert werden konnte bei verbesserter Effektivität in Kombination mit RBV (33, 34). Die Nebenwirkungsraten von PEG-IFN sind vergleichbar mit denen von Interferon-α (-2b). Die SVR-Raten von PEG-IFN und RBV liegen bei Patienten mit einer Genotyp-1-Infektion zwischen 38 und 49 % bei einer Therapiedauer von 48 Wochen (35).

Mit der Entschlüsselung des HCV-Genoms und neuer Replikationserkenntnisse konnten DAA entwickelt werden. Die DAA der ersten Generation wurden als sogenannte Trippeltherapien in Kombination mit PEG-IFN und RBV eingesetzt und haben zu einer kürzeren Therapiedauer und einer Erhöhung der Effektivitätsrate von bis zu 75 % der Genotyp-1-Behandlungen geführt. Allerdings sind diese Therapien mit starken Medikamenteninteraktionen und Nebenwirkungen verbunden und nur für die Behandlung von Genotyp-1-Infektionen einsetzbar gewesen (16, 36). Erst die Zulassung der DAA der zweiten Generation hat das Krankheitsmanagement für chronisch HCV-Infizierte grundlegend verändert. Mit diesen DAA stehen CHC-Erkrankten effiziente und nebenwirkungsärmere orale Therapiekombinationen bei kürzerer Therapiedauer zur Verfügung. Dieses gilt auch für therapieerfahrene Patienten und für solche mit fortgeschrittener Leberzirrhose, unabhängig vom Genotyp (27, 37). In Deutschland kann jeder CHC-Erkrankte grundsätzlich eine DAA-Therapie bekommen, es bestehen keine Restriktionen in Bezug auf den Grad der Leberschädigung (19). Die interferonfreien DAA-Therapien erreichen SVR-Raten von über 90 % bei einer Therapiedauer von acht oder zwölf, in Einzelfällen bis zu 24 Wochen (16, 27, 37, 38). Eine Therapie der CHC-Infektion gilt als erfolgreich, wenn die HCV-Viren-RNA zwölf Wochen nach Ende der Therapie nicht mehr im Blut nachweisbar ist (19, 37). Als Virennachweisgrenze gilt eine HCV-RNA <12-15 ml IU/ml, es müssen allerdings je nach Testsystem Unterschiede in den therapierelevanten Cut-offs berücksichtigt werden (19, 39). SVR sind mit einer Verringerung der HCV-verursachten Morbidität und Mortalität bei CHC-Kranken assoziiert und mit einer Verbesserung der Lebensqualität (40–43).

Die WHO hat die HCV-Infektion als weltweite Gefahr für die öffentliche Gesundheit bezeichnet und pangenotypische DAA 2017 in die Liste der unentbehrlichen Arzneimittel aufgenommen. Mit ihrer *Global Health Sector Strategy on Viral Hepatitis* verfolgt sie seit 2016 das Ziel, die Virushepatitis (B und C) bis zum Jahr 2030 zu eliminieren (44).

Die Hepatitis C als Berufskrankheit

Das Berufskrankheiten-Verfahren

Bei einem begründeten Verdacht auf das Vorliegen einer BK besteht für Ärzte eine Anzeigepflicht. Verdachtsanzeigen können auch andere Akteure wie Krankenkassen, Arbeitgeber oder Versicherte bei den Trägern der gesetzlichen Unfallversicherung (UV) stellen. Gemäß SGB VII, § 9 Abs. 1 ist eine BK eine Erkrankung, die ein Versicherter aufgrund seiner beruflichen Tätigkeit erleidet und die von der Bundesregierung durch Rechtsverordnung als BK bezeichnet wird. Hierunter zählen Krankheiten, „die nach den Erkenntnissen der medizinischen Wissenschaft durch be-sondere Einwirkungen verursacht sind, denen bestimmte Personengruppen durch ihre versicherte Tätigkeit in erheblich höherem Grade als die übrige Bevölkerung ausgesetzt sind (...)" (9). Krankheiten sind anerkennungsfähig als BK, wenn sie in der Anlage zur BK-Verordnung (BKV) aufgeführt sind oder wenn zum Entscheidungszeitpunkt nach neuen Erkenntnissen der medizinischen Wissenschaft die Voraussetzungen für eine Bezeichnung nach Absatz 1 erfüllt sind. Der UV-Träger prüft im Feststellungsverfahren, ob eine BK im Sinne der BKV vorliegt (§ 9 Abs. 1

und 2 (9)). Zwischen versicherter Tätigkeit und schädigender Einwirkung muss ein Zusammenhang im Vollbeweis bestehen, ebenso muss die Erkrankung im Vollbeweis vorliegen.

Die Aufgabe der UV ist die Verhütung von Arbeitsunfällen und BK sowie die Wiederherstellung der Gesundheit mit allen geeigneten Mitteln (45). Erst wenn die Möglichkeiten der Rehabilitation ausgeschöpft wurden und eine Minderung der Erwerbsfähigkeit (MdE) von mindestens 20 % länger als 26 Wochen besteht, wird eine BK als Versicherungsfall mit Rentenanspruch anerkannt (§ 56 Abs. 1 (46)). Die Höhe der Rentenleistung richtet sich nach der MdE des Versicherten (47). Diese wird im Rahmen eines Gutachterverfahrens nach dem Umfang der verminderten Arbeitsmöglichkeiten auf dem gesamten Gebiet des Erwerbslebens, die aus den körperlichen und geistigen Beeinträchtigungen in Folge der BK resultieren (§ 56 Abs. 2 (46)), eingeschätzt.

Beruflich verursachte HCV-Infektionen

HCV-Infektionen gehören zur dritten Gruppe (Infektionskrankheiten) der BK-Liste. Unter die BK Nummer 3101 fallen BK, die von Mensch zu Mensch übertragbar sind. Bei diesen Infektionskrankheiten ist der Nachweis des Ursachenzusammenhangs zwischen Einwirkung und Erkrankung sowie die Ermittlung des konkreten Infektionsvorgangs oftmals schwierig. Das Bundessozialgericht (BSG) hat die besondere Infektionsgefahr an die Stelle der Einwirkung bei der BK 3101 gesetzt (48). Für diese Krankheiten gilt der Vorbehalt, dass sie durch Tätigkeiten im Gesundheitsdienst verursacht wurden oder wenn ein vergleichbares Infektionsrisiko bestand (§ 9 Abs. 1 (9)).

Die Begutachtung der MdE erfolgt auf Grundlage morphologischer Kriterien, wie z. B. die Bestimmung der entzündlichen Aktivität (Grading) und des Fibroseausmaßes (Staging), sowie weiterer serologischer und klinischfunktioneller Untersuchungsergebnisse. In Abhängigkeit von der Stärke der Virenlast und der Leberschädigung wird der Grad der MdE eingestuft (*Tab. 1*) (49). Darüber hinaus wird im § 56 Abs. 2 (46) festgelegt, dass bei der Bemessung der MdE ebenfalls berufliche Nachteile zu berücksichtigen sind, die die Versicherten erleiden, dadurch dass ihnen Tätigkeitsfelder gemäß ihrer Qualifikation zum Schutz Dritter verschlossen bleiben (47).

Tabelle 1 „MdE-Bewertung der chronischen Hepatitis B und C im gutachterlichen Routinebetrieb der gesetzlichen Unfallversicherung" (49)

Entzündliche Aktivität	Fibrose			Zirrhose*
	null – gering	mäßig	stark	
gering	20 %	30 %	40 %	50 %
mäßig	30 %	40 %	50 %	60 %
stark	40 %	50 %	60 %	≥70 %

* Die klinischen Komplikationen sind zu berücksichtigen (portale Hypertension, Oesophagusvarizen (-blutung), Ascites, hepatische Enzephalopathie, primäres Leberzell-Ca) und erhöhen die MdE unter Umständen bis auf 100 %.

Dokumentation der BK-Meldungen

Die wesentlichen Merkmale einer BK-Verdachtsanzeige werden bei dem jeweils zuständigen UV-Träger standardisiert in einer Dokumentations-Datenbank (BK-DOK) erfasst. Wenn Hinweise auf eine Infektion vorliegen, werden Verdachtsanzeigen grundsätzlich als meldepflichtig erfasst.

Im Jahr 2016 waren über 44 % der angezeigten BK-Fälle bei der Berufsgenossenschaft für Gesundheitsdienst und Wohlfahrtspflege (BGW) Infektionskrankheiten im Sinne einer BK 3101. Am häufigsten stammten diese Verdachtsanzeigen aus Krankenhäusern und Kliniken (50).

Berufliche Exposition bei BiG

BiG arbeiten in Settings mit spezifischen Unfall- und Erkrankungsrisiken. Bei den blutübertragbaren Infektionskrankheiten ist vor allem der Kontakt zu infizierten Patienten bei invasiven Tätigkeiten, die mit einer erhöhten Verletzungsgefahr für die Beschäftigten einhergehen, von Bedeutung (6). Verletzungen des medizinischen Personals mit scharfen oder spitzen Gegenständen werden unter Nadelstichverletzungen (NSV) zusammenfasst und zählen zu den am häufigsten gemeldeten Arbeitsunfällen bei der BGW (51, 52). Ergebnisse aus epidemiologischen Studien weisen darauf hin, dass circa 80 % der BiG von NSV betroffen sind, die Dunkelziffer nicht gemeldeter NSV wird als erheblich eingeschätzt (7, 53). Die Identifizierung des Infektionszeitpunktes sowie des Indexpatienten ist aufgrund der fehlenden spezifischen Symptomatik der HCV-Infektion schwierig. Das Risiko einer Serokonversion hängt von der Art und Tiefe der Verletzung, der Menge des übertragenen infektiösen Materials und der Höhe der Viruslast des Indexpatienten ab (53–56). Die Wahrscheinlichkeit einer HCV-Serokonversion nach einer NSV wird in Europa mit 0,42 % als gering eingestuft (7, 53, 54).

Prävention

Derzeit stehen zur Prävention einer beruflich erworbenen HCV-Infektion nur Maßnahmen des technischen Infektionsschutzes zur Verfügung (57). Es existiert weder ein Impfstoff gegen den HCV-Virus noch eine Postexpositionsprophylaxe. Die Vermeidung von NSV als Schutz vor einer Infektion ist derzeit die wichtigste Präventionsmaßnahme. In dem 1999 in Kraft getretenen § 15 der Biostoffverordnung (BioStoffV (58)) wird auf Grundlage des Arbeitsschutzes die arbeitsmedizinische Vorsorge (ArbMedVV) geregelt. Gemäß der ArbMedVV besteht eine Pflichtvorsorgeuntersuchung bei Tätigkeiten mit erhöhter Infektionsgefährdung für HCV. Darüber hinaus werden in der BioStoffV die technischen Regeln vorgegeben, die den Umgang mit Gefährdungen bestimmen und Schutzmaßnahmen festlegen. Mit der EU-Richtlinie 2010/32 zur Vermeidung von NSV wurden verbindliche Mindestanforderungen zur Prophylaxe festgeschrieben und in der Novellierung der ArbMedVV von 2013 mit den Technischen Regeln für Biologische Arbeitsstoffe (TRBA 250 (59)) in nationales Recht umgesetzt. Darin wurden verbindliche Schutzmaßnahmen festgelegt, wie die Verwendung von stichsicheren Instrumenten (SSI) bei Tätigkeiten mit großer Infektionsgefährdung, der sichere Umgang mit spitzen und scharfen Instrumenten wie z. B. das Verbot von Recapping, und die ordnungsgemäße Entsorgung in ausschließlich dafür vorgesehenen Behältern (51).

Nach einer NSV soll neben der Meldung und Dokumentation eine direkte Risikoabschätzung vorgenommen werden. Ein Virusnachweis sofort nach einer NSV sollte gegebenenfalls zum Ausschluss einer bestehenden HCV-Infektion (bei unbekannten Status) und nach zwei bis sechs Wochen nach dem Ereignis erfolgen. Es wird der sichere Ausschluss einer Infektion durch einen zusätzlichen RNA-Nachweis gefordert, unter Berücksichtigung der maximal möglichen Inkubationszeit (60).

Nach den Daten der BGW sind die beruflich verursachten HCV-Infektionen rückläufig (*Abb. 2*). In den Jahren 1996 bis 2016 wurden insgesamt 3.380 entsprechende Anzeigen erfasst. Im selben Zeitraum wurde die Infektion bei 1.184 Versicherten als BK anerkannt. Über die Zeit betrachtet, ging die Anzahl der angezeigten und anerkannten Fälle um 77 % bzw. 83 % zurück.

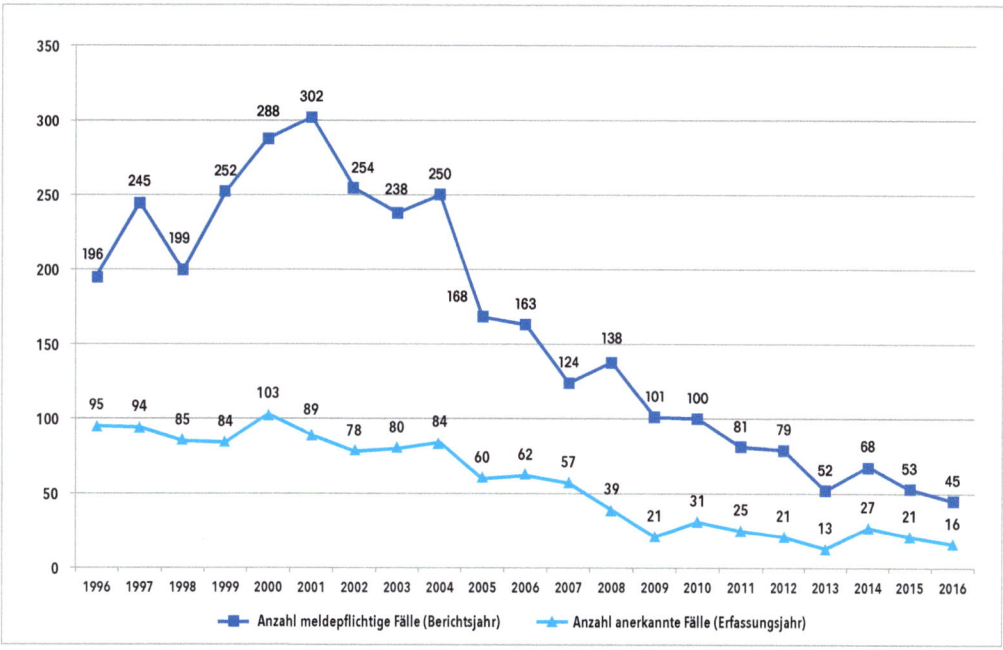

Abbildung 2 Entwicklung der meldepflichtigen Verdachtsanzeigen auf eine HCV und der anerkannten Fälle nach Erfassungs- bzw. Berichtsjahr (1996-2016; BGW-Daten)

Trotz der rückläufigen Zahlen ist die HCV im Gesundheitswesen weiterhin eine der häufigsten Infektion, die von der BGW als BK anerkannt wird. Sie ist ferner der häufigste Grund für eine neu bewilligte Rente (61).

Die vorliegende Arbeit besteht aus drei Publikationen zum Thema HCV bei BiG. Sie sind im Rahmen des PhD-Programms für Nichtmediziner an der Medizinischen Fakultät der Universität Hamburg am Universitätsklinikum Hamburg-Eppendorf (UKE) durchgeführt worden. Inhaltlich und methodisch beschäftigen sie sich mit dem Stand der Forschung zu relevanten Aspekten der HCV-Infektion als BK. In der ersten Studie wird die HCV-Betroffenheit bei BiG im Vergleich zu Kontrollen in Form einer Metaanalyse erstmalig quantitativ untersucht. Die gepoolte Analyse ist eine wichtige Voraussetzung zur Einschätzung der beruflichen Exposition. Sie ist für das BK-Feststellungsverfahren von besonderer Bedeutung, sowohl für die BGW als UV-Träger als auch für den einzelnen Beschäftigten. Der progrediente Krankheitsverlauf in Verbindung mit den jeweiligen Therapiemöglichkeiten hat zu hohen Entschädigungsleistungen durch die UV-Träger geführt. Die zweite Publikation befasst sich vor allem mit den Kosten der berufsbedingten CHC. Seit der Entwicklung der DAA-Medikamente lassen sich große Behandlungserfolge bei dieser

Krankheit beobachten. Die therapeutischen Erfolge der DAA-Therapien bei BiG werden in der dritten Publikation untersucht. Darüber hinaus wird untersucht, welche Auswirkungen die Behandlungsergebnisse auf die MdE der Beschäftigten haben.

1.3 Publikation 1 – Prävalenz der Hepatitis C bei Beschäftigten im Gesundheitswesen im Vergleich zur Allgemeinbevölkerung – Metaanalyse

1.3.1 Studienziel

Die Arbeit im Gesundheitswesen ist mit spezifischen Tätigkeiten verbunden, die für die Beschäftigten, die Kontakt zu infizierten Patienten und Blut haben, mit Gesundheitsrisiken einhergehen. Hervorzuheben sind in diesem Zusammenhang die wiederholt vorkommenden invasiven Tätigkeiten (exposure prone procedures), die eine potenzielle Verletzungsgefahr für die Beschäftigten darstellen (6). Die Übertragung des Hepatitis-C-RNA-Virus im beruflichen Kontext erfolgt über den Kontakt zu infektiösem Blut, verursacht durch eine NSV. Für die Beschäftigten kann eine HCV-Infektion schwerwiegende gesundheitliche, soziale, psychische und finanzielle Folgen haben (10). PEG-IFN-basierte Therapien sind über Jahrzehnte die Therapie der Wahl gewesen, mit langer Behandlungsdauer, mäßigen Erfolgsraten und mit zum Teil erheblichen Nebenwirkungen (10, 35). Statistisch gesehen ist eine beruflich erworbene HCV-Infektion selten, die damit einhergehenden Konsequenzen für die Betroffenen und für das Gesundheitssystem sind jedoch erheblich (53, 55, 62). Es gibt zahlreiche Studien zur Prävalenz von Hepatitis C bei BiG, die Ergebnisse zum Risiko einer HCV-Infektion sind jedoch inkonsistent. Anhand eines systematischen Reviews sollte untersucht werden, ob BiG im Vergleich zur Allgemeinbevölkerung aufgrund ihrer beruflichen Tätigkeiten ein erhöhtes HCV-Infektionsrisiko haben. Berufsgruppenspezifische Effektschätzer sollten ermittelt werden.

1.3.2 Methoden

Eine systematische Literaturrecherche wurde in den Datenbanken MEDLINE, EMBASE und COCHRANE LIBRARY für den Zeitraum von 1989 bis 2014 durchgeführt. Eingeschlossen wurden alle Prävalenz- und Inzidenzstudien zu Hepatitis C bei BiG mit serologischem Nachweis, die eine Kontrollgruppe oder Referenzdaten zur Allgemeinbevölkerung berücksichtigten. Die Suchstrings für die EMBASE-

Datenbank waren (((('hepatitis C') AND 'occupational exposure') AND 'healthcare worker') AND prevalence) OR incidence). Die Suchstrategie wurde für die anderen Datenbanken angepasst. Die eingeschlossenen Studien wurden nach ihrer methodischen Qualität bewertet.

Zur Einschätzung beruflicher Risiken wurde eine Metaanalyse durchgeführt. Es wurden Prävalenzraten sowie gepoolte Effektschätzer (Odds Ratios, OR) anhand der Mantel-Haenszel-Methode für dichotome Outcomes berechnet, angegeben werden diese mit einem 95%-Konfidenzintervall. Differenzierte Analysen wurden z. B. für Berufsgruppen und Kontrollen vorgenommen.

1.3.3 Ergebnisse

Insgesamt wurden 3.016 Publikationen in den Datenbanken und weitere 41 über die Handrecherche identifiziert. In das systematische Review wurden 57 Studien eingeschlossen, 44 davon konnten in der Metaanalyse berücksichtigt werden. Die Studien stammen hautsächlich aus Europa (n = 27) und Asien (n = 13), wenige aus Afrika (n = 8), Nordamerika (n = 7) und Südamerika (n = 2). Die untersuchten Outcomes variieren stark, die Beschäftigten wurden nur in wenigen Studien stratifiziert nach Berufsgruppen (n = 5) oder nach Exposition (n = 5) untersucht. Die gepoolte HCV-Prävalenz wurde mit 1,1% (95%-CI 0,92-1,32) für die BiG und 0,6% (95%-CI 0,48-0,72) für die Kontrollen berechnet.

Die gepoolte Analyse der methodisch guten und moderaten Studien mit Bestätigungstests ergab ein statistisch signifikant erhöhtes OR für eine HCV-Infektion bei BiG im Vergleich zur Allgemeinbevölkerung (OR 1,6; 95%-CI 1,03-2,42). Die Stratifizierung nach Ländern mit vergleichbar niedriger HCV-Prävalenz in Europa (Belgien, Dänemark, Frankreich, Schottland, Schweden) und den USA ergab ein OR von 2,1 (95%-CI 1,31-3,42) für die BiG im Vergleich zu den Kontrollen insgesamt. Die Analyse für Berufsgruppen zeigt im Vergleich zur Allgemeinbevölkerung ein größeres Infektionsrisiko für Ärzte (OR 2,7; 95%-CI 1,65-4,51) und für BiG, die ein großes Risiko für Blutkontakte aufgrund invasiver Tätigkeiten haben (OR 2,7; 95%-CI 1,65-4,25; *Abb. 3*). Die Stratifizierung für das Laborpersonal ergab ein OR von 2,2 (95%-CI 1,10-4,39) im Vergleich zu den Kontrollen insgesamt (*Abb. 3*). Für das Pflegepersonal ergab die gepoolte Analyse ein OR von 1,7 (95%-CI 0,86-3,31) im Vergleich zu populationsbezogenen Kontrollen.

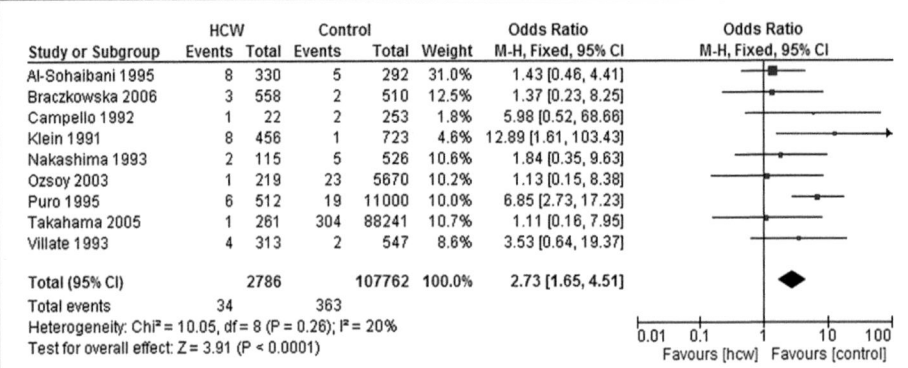

Strata: ärztliches Personal im Vergleich zu populationsbezogenen Kontrollen

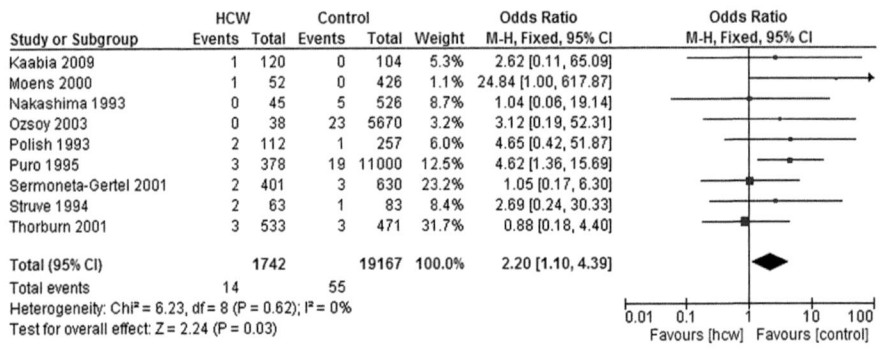

Strata: Labormitarbeiter im Vergleich zu Kontrollen insgesamt

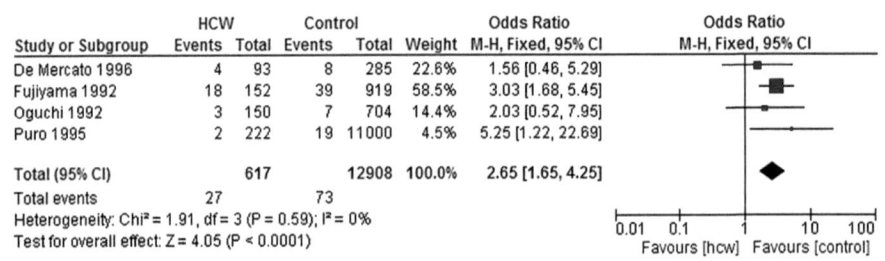

Strata: BIG mit hohem Risiko für Blutkontakte im Vergleich zu populationsbezogenen Kontrollen

Legende: HCW = BiG (Beschäftigte im Gesundheitswesen), Control = Kontrollen

Abbildung 3 Forest Plots der methodisch guten und moderaten Studien mit HCV-Bestätigungstests

1.3.4 Diskussion

Die Ergebnisse dieser Metaanalyse zeigen für BiG ein statistisch signifikant erhöhtes OR von 1,6 (95%-CI 1,03-2,42) für eine HCV-Infektion im Vergleich zur Allgemeinbevölkerung. Ein wesentliches Ergebnis der Analyse sind die gepoolten Effektschätzer für die BiG, differenziert nach Beruf oder Exposition. Als signifikant exponiert erwiesen sich das ärztliche und das Laborpersonal ebenso wie die BiG, die ein hohes Risiko für Blutkontakte aufgrund der Durchführung invasiver Tätigkeiten haben. Für das Pflegepersonal ergab die gepoolte Analyse kein signifikant erhöhtes Infektionsrisiko. Eine differenzierte Betrachtung der Exposition aufgrund von spezifischen Tätigkeitsprofilen wurde vor allem für diese Beschäftigtengruppe nur unzureichend durchgeführt. Diese mangelnde Differenzierung führt zu einer möglichen Unterschätzung des beruflichen Infektionsrisikos aufgrund einer Missklassifikation der Exposition. Dieses findet insbesondere statt, wenn Beschäftigte, die eine starke berufliche Exposition gegenüber Blutkontakten bei gleichzeitigem Umgang mit verletzungsträchtigen scharfen Instrumenten haben, zusammen mit Beschäftigten untersucht werden, bei denen dies nicht der Fall ist. Blutkontakte, hervorgerufen durch NSV, stellen eine Gefahr einer berufsbedingten HCV-Infektion für BiG dar. Im Sinne der Prävention einer beruflich erworbenen Infektion ist ein gut zugängliches Melde- und Behandlungssystem eine ebenso notwendige Voraussetzung wie die Kenntnis und Anwendung von sicheren Verfahrensweisen und Instrumenten.

1.4 Publikation 2 – Kosten und Trends für beruflich bedingte Hepatitis-C-Infektionen

1.4.1 Studienziel

Ein Großteil der HCV-Infektionen verläuft ohne klinisch optische Symptome und bleibt mit einer Chronifizierungsrate von bis zu 85 % häufig unentdeckt. Die CHC-Infektion ist aufgrund ihrer Progredienz und der in der Vergangenheit fehlenden adäquaten Behandlungsmöglichkeiten mit hohen Morbiditäts- und Mortalitätsraten assoziiert (1, 20, 22). Sie ist ein Risikofaktor für die Entwicklung eines Leber-zellkarzinoms, das in der Rangfolge der krebsbedingten Todesfälle weltweit den zweiten Platz einnimmt und die Hauptindikation für eine viral bedingte Lebertransplantation ist (2, 3). Der chronische Verlauf geht einher mit einer Minderung der gesundheitsbezogenen Lebensqualität der Betroffenen und mit neuropsychiatrischen Symptomen, die durch Interferon-alpha-Behandlungen verstärkt werden Solche

Symptome können zu erheblichen Beeinträchtigungen für den Betroffenen führen, ohne dass eine organische Beeinträchtigung der Leber vorliegt (10, 63). Als Ursache für kognitive Beeinträchtigungen werden direkte Auswirkungen der HCV-Infektion auf das Zentralnervensystem vermutet (64). Die ökonomische Relevanz der CHC-Infektion ergibt sich aus den Krankheitsfolgen und den daraus resultierenden Behandlungskosten sowie aus Produktivitätsverlusten durch Arbeits- und Erwerbsunfähigkeit (65). US-amerikanische Wissenschaftler haben die CHC-assoziierten Kosten von 53.796 Patienten mit CHC aus den Jahren 2002 bis 2010 anhand von Daten einer privaten Krankenversicherung berechnet. Die durchschnittlichen Kosten betrugen je Patient und Jahr circa 21.776 Euro. Stratifiziert nach Krankheitsstadien waren sie am höchsten bei Patienten mit terminaler Leberzirrhose (53.880 Euro pro Patient jährlich) (62). Aufgrund des potenziell schweren Krankheitsverlaufs und der hohen assoziierten Kosten liegt die erfolgreiche Behandlung der CHC im Interesse der sozialen Sicherungssysteme (31, 62). Mit den DAA der zweiten Generation stehen heute vielversprechende Therapiekombinationen zur Verfügung. Ziel dieser Arbeit ist es, die Kosten für die beruflich bedingten Hepatitis-C-Infektionen anhand der Daten der BGW für den Zeitraum von 2000 bis 2014 zu beschreiben.

1.4.2 Methoden

Für die Auswertung wurden die Routinedaten der BGW verwendet. Als Datenquelle diente die BK-DOK. Die Analyse basiert auf Daten von Versicherten, deren HCV-Infektionen zwischen 1996 und 2013 als BK anerkannt wurden. Der Grad der MdE bildet die Grundlage für die Rentenleistung. Die Daten zu Entschädigungsleistungen werden erst seit 2000 erfasst und aufbereitet. Berücksichtigt haben wir die Buchungen, die zwischen dem 1.1.2000 und dem 31.12.2014 getätigt wurden. Die Buchungstitel wurden gruppiert und auf neun Kategorien reduziert. Die Ergebnisse werden deskriptiv dargestellt (absolute Häufigkeiten) und die angefallenen Kosten werden über den Beobachtungszeitraum von 15 Jahren aufsummiert.

1.4.3 Ergebnisse

In den Jahren 1996 bis 2013 wurden bei der BGW insgesamt 3.230 Anzeigen auf Verdacht einer beruflich bedingten Infektion mit HCV erfasst. Im selben Zeitraum wurde die Infektion bei 1.121 Versicherten als BK anerkannt. Über die Zeit betrachtet ging die Anzahl der angezeigten und anerkannten Fälle um 73 % bzw. 86 % zurück.

Zum Zeitpunkt der Erfassung der BK-Anzeige waren von den 1.121 Versicherten mit einer beruflich bedingten HCV-Infektion 75 % weiblich, insgesamt waren knapp 70 % älter als 40 Jahre. Der größte Anteil der Versicherten war in Krankenhäusern beschäftigt (46 %) und über 90 % übten zur Zeit der Erkrankung eine medizinisch-pflegerische Tätigkeit aus (*Tab.2*).

Tabelle 2 Beschreibung der Stichprobe von Versicherten mit einer anerkannten Hepatitis-C-Infektion nach soziodemografischen Merkmalen (n = 1.121)

Merkmale	N	%
Geschlecht, weiblich	838	75
Alter (Jahre)*		
< 20	17	1
21–40	335	30
41–60	646	58
> 61	123	11
Tätigkeitsbereich		
Klinik/Krankenhaus	510	46
Arztpraxen	341	30
Alten- und Krankenpflege	131	12
Ambulant-sozialpflegerischer Dienst	79	7
Verwaltung	60	5

*Alter zum Stichtag (31.12.2014)

Am häufigsten wurde die erste MdE mit 20 % eingestuft. Nur vereinzelt gab es Fälle mit einer ersten MdE von 100 %. In 57 % der Fälle gab es keine Erhöhung der MdE über die Dauer der Erkrankung. Die Rentenansprüche auf Basis einer vorliegenden MdE von 60 % und höher entfielen zum Stichtag zu 88 % auf Versicherte, deren BK-Meldung vor 2005, bzw. zu 100 % auf Versicherte, deren BK-Meldung bis 2010 erfolgte.

Entwicklung der Ausgaben

Die aufsummierten Entschädigungsleistungen für den Zeitraum von 2000 bis 2014 betrugen 87,9 Millionen Euro. Davon entfielen knapp 60 % auf Rentenzahlungen und circa 15 % auf Ausgaben für Arznei- und Heilmittel.

Über den 15-jährigen Beobachtungszeitraum haben sich die Entschädigungs-
leistungen für medizinische (Heil- und Arzneimittel) und berufliche Rehabilitation
(Wiedereingliederung, Umschulungen) sowie für Renten unterschiedlich entwickelt
(*Abb. 4*). Die jährlichen Aufwendungen sind zwischen 2000 und 2005 von 2,6 konti-
nuierlich auf 6,3 Millionen Euro angestiegen. Zwischen 2005 und 2010 lagen sie bei
6 Millionen Euro jährlich, stiegen im Jahr 2012 auf 7,3 und auf 8,3 Millionen Euro im
Jahr 2014. Mit Ausnahme des Jahres 2014 machten die Leistungen für medizinische
Rehabilitation etwa ein Drittel und die Aufwendungen für Renten etwa zwei Drittel
der jährlichen Kosten aus. Im Jahr 2014 beliefen sich die Ausgaben für medizinische
Rehabilitation auf etwa die Hälfte der Ausgaben insgesamt. Die Ausgaben für
Rentenleistungen stiegen von 1,6 Millionen Euro im Jahr 2000 kontinuierlich bis auf
über 4 Millionen Euro im Jahr 2014. Die Ausgaben für Leistungen zur Teilhabe am
Arbeitsleben (berufliche Rehabilitation) lagen in allen Jahren unter 1% der Gesamt-
ausgaben.

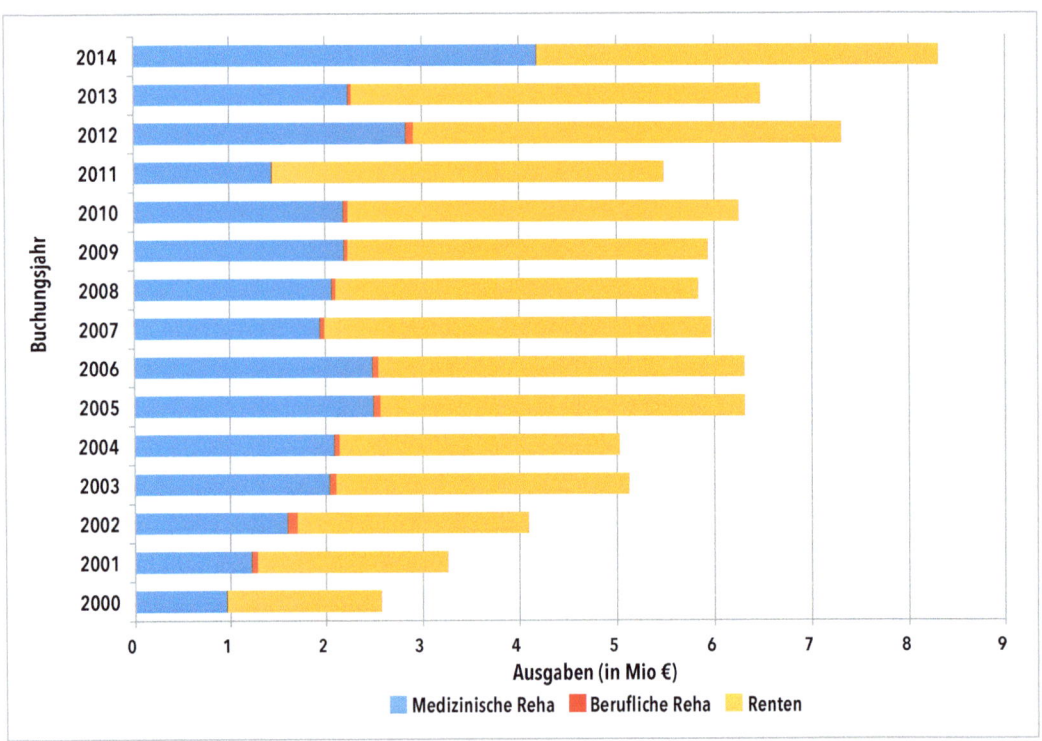

Abbildung 4 Leistungen für medizinische, berufliche Rehabilitation und Rentenzahlungen
für anerkannte HCV-Fälle bei insgesamt 1.097 Fällen in den Jahren 2000 bis 2014

Medikamente zur Therapie der Hepatitis C

Die Ausgaben für Medikamente sind von 255.730 Euro im Jahr 2000 kontinuierlich auf rund 1 Million Euro im Jahr 2005 angestiegen, in den Folgejahren bis 2010 lagen sie unter 800.000 Euro (*Abb. 5*). Ein deutlicher Anstieg bei den Ausgaben für Medikamente gab es in den Jahren 2012 und 2014. Im Vergleich zu den jährlichen Kosten, die für die Jahre 2005 bis 2010 angefallen sind, beträgt der Kostenanstieg für Medikamente im Jahr 2012 über 70 % und im Jahr 2014 über 120 %

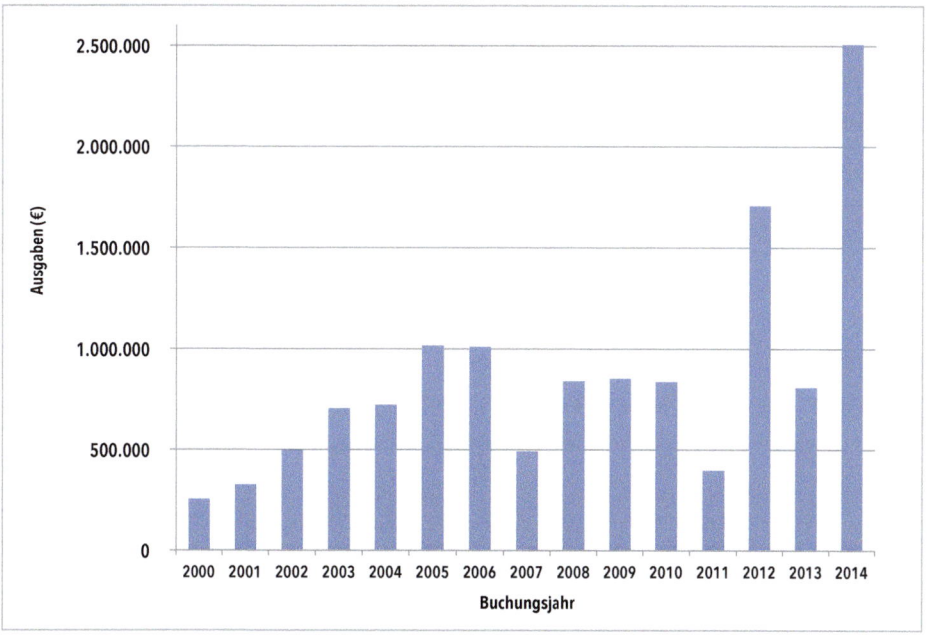

Abbildung 5 Ausgaben für Medikamente für die Stichprobe anerkannter HCV-Fälle, aufgeführt nach Buchungsjahr

1.4.4 Diskussion

Für die HCV-Infektion als BK ist ein anhaltend rückläufiger Trend sowohl bei der Anzahl der gemeldeten Verdachts- als auch bei den anerkannten BK-Fällen zu beobachten, bei gleichzeitig steigenden Kosten. Die Kosten für die CHC wurden überwiegend von den steigenden Ausgaben für Rentenleistungen bestimmt. Die Renten für beruflich bedingte CHC erklären 60 % der Kosten, die in den Jahren 2000 bis 2014 insgesamt für die untersuchten BK-Fälle aufgebracht wurden. In den Jahren 2012 und 2014 gab es jeweils einen starken Anstieg der Kosten für die medikamentöse Therapie. Der Anstieg der Kosten im Jahr 2012 auf 1,7 Millionen Euro in der untersuchten Stichprobe lässt sich wahrscheinlich auf die Ausgaben für die Behandlung mit Triplekombinationen aus PEG-IFN, RBV und einem Proteaseinhibitor der ersten Generation zurückführen. Der Anstieg bei den Ausgaben für Medikamente im Jahr 2014 auf 2,5 Millionen Euro geht vermutlich auf den Einsatz von DAA der zweiten Generation zurück. Die DAA-Regime erreichen bei kürzeren und in der Tendenz nebenwirkungsärmeren Therapien hohe SVR-Raten (66). Gemäß Nevens und Kollegen (2012) reduzierten sich die Kosten nach erfolgreicher Therapie für die Versorgung von CHC-Erkrankten (Genotyp 1) mit kompensierter Leberzirrhose um 45 % im Beobachtungszeitraum von drei Jahren (67). SVR sind mit einer Verringerung der CHC-verursachten (hepatischen und extrahepatischen) Morbidität und Mortalität assoziiert (40, 43). Es wurden funktionelle Verbesserungen der Leberzirrhose nach Erreichen von SVR beobachtet sowie anhaltende Erfolge in der Behandlung von extrahepatischen Manifestationen (66, 68). Die präoperative Behandlung mit dem Ziel einer SVR zum Zeitpunkt der Transplantation reduziert nachhaltig das Risiko einer Reinfektion mit HCV (40, 69). Die Diagnosestellung zu einem frühen Zeitpunkt der HCV-Infektion ist ein wichtiger Faktor, um eine möglichst vollständige Heilung zu erreichen. Langfristig lassen sich voraussichtlich die hohen Kosten der Therapie dadurch amortisieren, dass durch eine frühe Heilung von CHC-Infektionen Morbiditäts- und Mortalitätsraten verringert werden.

1.5 Publikation 3 – Hepatitis C bei Beschäftigten im Gesundheitswesen: Sekundärdatenanalyse zu den Therapien mit direkt antiviral wirksamen Medikamenten

1.5.1 Studienziel

Mit den DAA stehen CHC-Infizierten effiziente orale Therapiekombinationen zur Verfügung, unabhängig vom Grad der Leberschädigung und des Genotyps. Im Gesundheitswesen ist die Hepatitis C, trotz rückläufiger Zahlen, weiterhin eine der häufigsten Infektionen, die zu einer BK-Anerkennung und zu einer BK-Rente führen (61). Die Analyse der Daten der BGW zeigen, dass zwar die Inzidenz von berufsbedingten HCV-Infektionen in den vergangenen Jahren stetig zurückgegangen ist, die Kosten insgesamt allerdings deutlich angestiegen sind. Diese Kosten werden hauptsächlich durch den Anstieg der Kosten für Medikamente zur Behandlung der Infektion sowie durch den Anstieg der Entschädigungsleistungen für BK-Renten verursacht (70). Den hohen Kosten einer DAA-Therapie steht ein potenziell großer Nutzen gegenüber. Am Beispiel der beruflich bedingten CHC sollen die Behandlungsergebnisse der neuen DAA-Therapien bei BiG und deren Auswirkungen auf die MdE untersucht werden.

1.5.2 Methoden

Die Ergebnisanalyse der DAA-Therapien wurde anhand der Daten der BGW durchgeführt. In die Auswertung eingeschlossen wurden die anonymisierten Daten der Versicherten, die zwischen dem 1.1.2014 und dem 30.11.2016 eine DAA-Therapie abgeschlossen haben und bei denen die Ergebnisse der Therapie zwölf Wochen nach Therapieende vorlagen. Bei Therapieversagen direkt nach Therapieende wurde bei fehlenden Angaben zwölf Wochen nach Therapieende ebenfalls ein Therapieversagen angenommen. Als Relapse gilt ein Viren-RNA-Nachweis zwölf Wochen nach Therapieende nach vorherigen SVR (ETR, End of Treatment Response, Erfolgsrate direkt nach Therapieende). Mittels multivariater Regressionsanalyse wurden mögliche Zusammenhänge zwischen den Prädiktoren Zirrhose, Therapiestatus, Geschlecht sowie Alter (als stetiges Merkmal) und dem Erreichen von SVR zwölf Wochen nach Therapieende (SVR12) untersucht. Die untersuchten Endpunkte sind die Erfolgskontrollen (SVR12), die dokumentierten Therapienebenwirkungen sowie die Ergebnisse der Begutachtung der MdE nach der DAA-Therapie.

1.5.3 Ergebnisse

Die Stichprobe (n = 180) bestand zu 74 % aus Frauen, das Durchschnittsalter der Versicherten betrug 62 Jahre. Eine HCV-Genotyp-1-Infektion hatten 90 % der Versicherten, vereinzelt wurde die Infektion durch Viren des Genotyps 2 und 3 (je 4 %) bzw. 4 (<1 %) verursacht. Es wurden keine Komorbiditäten mit HBV- oder HIV-Infektionen angegeben. Vor Beginn der DAA-Therapie hatten 76 % der Versicherten einen Leberbefund (Fibrose 43 %, kompensierte bzw. dekompensierte Zirrhose 24 % bzw. 9 %), 72 % waren therapieerfahren. Eine MdE hatten über 90 % der Versicherten.

DAA-Behandlungsregime und dokumentierte Nebenwirkungen (Tab. 3)
Die am häufigsten durchgeführte DAA-Kombinationstherapie bestand aus Ledipasvir (LDV) und Sofosbuvir (SOF) (49 %). Eine DAA-Therapie mit RBV wurde in 20 %, die Kombination mit PEG-IFN und RBV in 2 % der Fälle angewendet. Die Therapiedauer lag zwischen acht und 24 Wochen, überwiegend bei zwölf Wochen

(71%). Bei 66% der Versicherten verlief die Therapie ohne Nebenwirkungen. Am häufigsten wurde als Nebenwirkung eine Kombination aus Symptomen wie Kopfschmerzen, Übelkeit, Schlafstörungen und Müdigkeit (26%) in hauptsächlich milder Ausprägung angegeben. Über Hautreaktionen wie Juckreiz bis hin zu generalisiertem Hautausschlag und phototoxische Reaktionen klagten 4% der Versicherten. Vereinzelt kam es zu Hämoglobinabfällen, Gefühlen von Angst, Reizbarkeit bis hin zu Depressionen sowie zu isolierten gastrointestinalen Beschwerden.

Tabelle 3 Angaben zu den DAA-Therapien (n=180)

Merkmal (fehlende Werte n/%)	Gültige Werte	
	n	%
Therapien gesamt (2/1)		
LDV,SOF	88	49
SOF, DCV	29	16
LDV, SOF, RBV	17	10
SOF, SMV	11	6
DSV, OBV, PTV, RTV, RBV	11	6
DSV, OBV, PTV, RTV	9	5
SOF, RBV	7	4
SOF, RBV, PEG-IFN	3	2
DCV, SOF, RBV	1	<1
SOF, SMV, RBV	1	<1
PEG-IFN, TVR, RBV	1	<1
Therapieergebnis		
Direkt nach Therapie		
ETR	173	97
Remission	6	3
zwölf Wochen nach Therapie		
SVR12	170	94
Remission/Viruslast unverändert	6	<3
Relapse	4	<3

DAA = direkt antiviral wirksame Medikamente; LDV = Ledipasvir; SOF = Sofosbuvir; DCV = Daclatasvir; RBV = Ribavirin; RTV = Ritonavir; SMV = Simeprevir; DSV = Dasabuvir; OBV = Ombitasvir; PTV = Paritaprevir; PEG-IFN = PEG-Interferon; TVR = Telaprevir; ETR = End of Treatment Response, SVR12 = sustained virological response zwölf Wochen nach Therapieende

Erfolgskontrollen und Ergebnisse der DAA-Therapien

Die ETR-Rate der untersuchten DAA-Regime betrug 97%, die SVR12-Rate 94% (*Tab.3*). Bei jeweils sechs Versicherten wurde direkt sowie zwölf Wochen nach Therapieende keine SVR erreicht, bei vier Versicherten kam es zu einem Relapse. Der Umstand, therapieerfahren gewesen zu sein, ergab im Gruppenvergleich keinen signifikanten Unterschied bei den SVR12-Raten (SVR12 98% versus 94%, p=0,44), beim Zirrhosestatus war der Unterschied statistisch signifikant (*Tab. 4*). Bei Versicherten ohne Leberzirrhose war die DAA-Therapie statistisch signifikant häufiger erfolgreich als bei Versicherten mit diagnostizierter Leberzirrhose (SVR12 98% versus 86%, p=0,006). Bei Versicherten mit einem MdE-Grad von 50% oder weniger war die DAA-Therapie ebenfalls signifikant häufiger erfolgreich als bei Versicherten mit einem MdE-Grad von mehr als 50% (SVR12 97% versus 86%, p=0,019). Frauen haben etwas häufiger eine SVR12 erreicht als Männer (nicht statistisch signifikant). In der multivariaten Regression zeigte sich, dass die Variablen Zirrhose und Alter in einem signifikanten Zusammenhang mit dem Erreichen von SVR12 standen. Versicherte mit einer Leberzirrhose hatten eine um zwölf Prozentpunkte geringere Chance eine SVR12 zu erreichen als Versicherte ohne eine Leberzirrhose. Dieser Effekt wurde bestätigt und war weiterhin signifikant. Mit steigendem Alter erhöht sich die Chance für das Erreichen von SVR12 im untersuchten Kollektiv (OR 1,11; 95%-CI 1,01-1,23, p=0,04). Die Variablen Vortherapiestatus und Geschlecht wiesen in der multivariaten Analyse keinen statistisch signifikanten Einfluss auf das Erreichen von SVR12 im Kollektiv auf. Zum Zeitpunkt der Auswertung lagen die Laborwerte der Leberenzyme (GOT, GPT, γGT) von 102 Versicherten zwölf Wochen nach Therapieende vor. Bei 90 Versicherten (88%) waren die Leberenzyme zwölf Wochen nach der DAA-Therapie im Normbereich.

Begutachtung der MdE nach DAA-Therapie (Tab. 4)

Eine Begutachtung der MdE nach der DAA-Therapie fand bei 115 Versicherten (64%) statt, im Mittel neun Monate nach Therapieende. Bei 76% (87 von 115) der Versicherten wurde die MdE angepasst. Dabei entfiel für 56 Versicherte die vor der Therapie festgelegte MdE, für 25 ergab das Gutachten eine Herab- sowie für sechs Versicherte eine Heraufstufung. Gründe für eine Heraufstufung waren: erfolgte Lebertransplantation nach erfolgreich vorangegangener DAA-Therapie, Ösophagusvarizen-Blutungen sowie ein beginnendes hepatorenales Syndrom.

Tabelle 4 Univariate und multivariate logistische Regressionsanalyse – Prädiktoren für SVR12 (n = 180)

Univariate Untersuchung					
Variable[a]	Fehlende Werte	n gesamt	% SVR12-Raten	OR (95%-CI)	p-Wert
Zirrhosestatus (nein/ja)	28	152 (102/50)	98% versus 86%	0,12 (0,03-0,62)	0,006
Therapiestatus (naiv/erfahren)	21	159 (45/114)	98% versus 94%	0,35 (0,04-2,90)	0,44
MdE[a] (≤50 %/>50 %)	5	175 (139/36)	97% versus 86%	0,18 (0,05-0,72)	0,02
Geschlecht (Frauen/Männer)	0	180 (133/47)	96% versus 88%	0,32 (0,09-1,19)	0,13

Multivariates logistisches Regressionsmodel mit Zielgröße SVR12					
Variable[a]	Fehlende Werte	n gesamt	OR (95%-CI)	p-Wert	R^2
Zirrhosestatus (nein/ja)	34	146 (98/48)	0,098 (0,01-0,75)	0,03	
Therapiestatus (naiv/erfahren)	34	146 (42/104)	0,42 (0,05-3,92)	0,42	0,242
Geschlecht (Frauen/Männer)	34	146 (112/34)	0,41 (0,08-2,18)	0,30	
Alter	34	146	1,11 (1,01-1,23)	0,04	

SVR12 = sustained virological response zwölf Wochen nach Therapieende;
MdE =Minderung der Erwerbsfähigkeit; a bei kategorialen Variablen wurde die erste Kategorie als Referenz
festgelegt; OR = Odds Ratio für die primäre Zielgröße SVR12

1.5.4 Diskussion

Im untersuchten Versichertenkollektiv erreichten CHC-Infizierte hohe SVR12-Raten (94%) durch die DAA-Therapien. Einen signifikanten Zusammenhang mit dem Therapieerfolg zwölf Wochen nach Therapieende wiesen der Zirrhosestatus und das Alter der Versicherten auf. Eine Leberzirrhose führte zu einer statistisch signifikant geringeren SVR12-Rate. Der Zusammenhang zwischen dem Alter der behandelten Versicherten und dem Erreichen von SVR12 ist ebenfalls signifikant. Die untersuchte Stichprobe hat ein mittleres Alter von 62 Jahren, eine Verzerrung des Alterseffekts ist nicht auszuschließen. Ein fortgeschrittenes Alter ist kein Hindernis für eine DAA-Therapieindikation. Weder die Therapieerfahrung noch das

Geschlecht standen in einem signifikanten Zusammenhang mit der Zielvariablen SVR12. Gemäß Zeuzem (72) bedeutet der fehlende Nachweis von HCV-RNA zwölf Wochen nach Ende der DAA-Therapie eine dauerhafte Viruseradikation. Rückfälle nach diesem Zeitpunkt seien selten, in der Regel handle es sich um Neuinfektionen.

Die im untersuchten Kollektiv am häufigsten eingesetzte DAA-Kombinations-therapie mit LDV und SOF (49 %) wurde gemäß Zimmermann und Kollegen (71) ebenfalls 2015 am häufigsten bei gesetzlich Krankenversicherten in Deutschland durchgeführt (64 %). Die Häufigkeit der Kombination mit RBV wurde in der Studie nicht quantifiziert. Für die (monatlichen) PEG-IFN-Therapie-Regime geben die Autoren einen Verschreibungsrückgang von ca. 2.700 im Januar 2014 auf circa 650 im Dezember 2015 an. In der vorliegenden Untersuchung wurde eine DAA-Therapie mit RBV in 36 Fällen (20 %), die Kombination mit PEG-IFN und RBV in vier Fällen (2 %) angewendet. Überwiegend dauerten die eingesetzten DAA-Regime zwölf Wochen (67 %). Vergleichbare Therapiezeiten werden in der German Hepatitis Co-hort (GECCO) beobachtet (72). Die in unserer Untersuchung am häufigsten beob-achteten Nebenwirkungen wie Übelkeit, Kopfschmerzen und Schlafstörungen führt auch Zeuzem (71) bei Therapien mit SOF und Semiprevir (SMV) an. Hämo-globinabfälle traten bei zwei DAA-Behandlungen (Versicherte mit Zirrhose) mit LDV und SOF in Kombination mit RBV auf. Das Auftreten von hämolytischer Anämie als Folge von Ribaviringabe wird in der Literatur beschrieben. Ferner wurden Nebenwirkungen wie Angst und Depression bei zwei vortherapierten Versicherten ohne Zirrhose beobachtet, die DAA kombiniert mit PEG-IFN oder RBV bekommen haben. Sowohl bei PEG-IFN als auch bei RBV und insbesondere in Kombination wird in der Literatur das Auftreten von Depressionen angegeben (73, 74). Die Therapien konnten ohne Unterbrechung erfolgreich durchgeführt werden (SVR12).

SVR sind mit einer Verringerung der CHC-verursachten Morbidität und Mortalität bei CHC-Kranken unabhängig vom Zirrhosestatus und mit einer Verbesserung der gesundheitsbezogenen Lebensqualität assoziiert (40-43). Im untersuchten Kollektiv zeigten sich im Mittel bereits neun Monate nach erfolgreicher Therapie positive Auswirkungen auf die Arbeitsfähigkeit der Versicherten. Eine Begutachtung wurde bei 115 Versicherten nach erfolgreicher DAA-Therapie durchgeführt, dabei wurde eine Verbesserung der MdE bei mehr als 70 % festgestellt. Da sich die Entwicklung der Rentenansprüche proportional zum Grad der MdE der Betroffenen verhält, ist in Zukunft mit geringeren Aufwendungen für Rentenzahlungen im Kollektiv zu rechnen. Das wichtigste Ergebnis dieser Studie ist der große therapeutische Erfolg

(SVR12 94 %), obwohl die Mehrheit der Versicherten bereits eine Leberschädigung hatte. Eine frühe Therapie ist erstrebenswert, um die individuelle Krankheitslast möglichst gering zu halten. Sie scheint auch aus Kostengründen indiziert, z. B. aufgrund des Einflusses des Zirrhosestatus auf den Therapieerfolg.

1.6 Diskussion

Über die Rolle der HCV-Infektion im Gesundheitswesen wurde lange Zeit infektionsepidemiologisch kontrovers diskutiert. Die Abgrenzung der beruflich erworbenen HCV-Infektion im BK-Anerkennungsverfahren stellte alle Akteure im Gesundheitswesen über Jahrzehnte vor eine schwierige Aufgabe. Aufgrund des wiederholten Kontakts zu möglicherweise infektiösen Körperflüssigkeiten war für die Beschäftigten von einem Risiko für eine beruflich bedingte Infektion auszugehen. Die Übertragungswahrscheinlichkeit von HCV wird als gering beschrieben und aufgrund ihres inapparenten Verlaufs wird die Infektion eher zufällig entdeckt. Die Übertragungsumstände sind aufgrund des nicht bekannten Infektionszeitpunkts schwierig bis kaum zu rekonstruieren und das konkrete Ereignis selten zu identifizieren. Für die BiG stellte diese Situation häufig eine Hürde im Prozess der BK-Anerkennung dar. Systematische Daten zur Prävalenz von Anti-HCV für BiG liegen aus Deutschland, Österreich und der Schweiz nicht vor (19). Die Metaanalyse zur Prävalenz der HCV bei BiG untersucht als erste Studie im Rahmen dieser Dissertation die Frage des beruflichen Ursachenzusammenhangs zwischen den ausgeführten Tätigkeiten und der Infektion mit HCV. Ihre Ergebnisse erlauben mit Einschränkungen eine differenzierte Betrachtung des beruflichen Risikos von medizinischem Personal für eine HCV-Infektion. Sie wird in der aktualisierten Fassung der S3-Leitlinie zur HCV-Infektion „Prophylaxe, Diagnostik und Therapie der Arbeitsgemeinschaft Wissenschaftlich Medizinischer Fachgesellschaften (AWMF)" in Zusammenhang mit einem beruflich bedingten Infektionsrisiko für BiG aufgeführt (19). Die Ergebnisse zeigen Unterschiede in der beruflichen Exposition aufgrund spezifischer Tätigkeitsprofile der Beschäftigten auf. Als signifikant exponiert im Vergleich zur Allgemeinbevölkerung erweisen sich die Beschäftigten, die ein hohes Risiko für Blutkontakte aufgrund der Durchführung invasiver Tätigkeiten haben (OR 2,7; 95%-CI 1,65-4,25). Berufsspezifisch konnte sowohl für das ärztliche als auch für das Laborpersonal ein signifikant erhöhtes OR von 2,7 beziehungsweise 2,2 für den Erwerb einer HCV-Infektion im Vergleich zu Kontrollen gezeigt werden. Für das Pflegepersonal wurde eine differenzierte Betrachtung der Exposition nach Tätigkeitsprofilen nur unzureichend durchgeführt. Für diese Beschäftigtengruppe, die mit zur größten im Gesundheitswesen zählt, führt die mangelnde Differenzierung zu einer möglichen Unterschätzung des beruflichen Infektionsrisikos aufgrund einer Missklassifikation der Exposition. Die Ergebnisse für die BiG insgesamt, unabhängig vom Tätigkeitsprofil und der Berufsgruppe, zeigen ein statistisch signifikant erhöhtes OR von 1,6 (95%-CI 1,03-2,42) für eine HCV-Infektion im Vergleich zur Allgemeinbevölkerung.

Im BK-Verfahren spielen die HCV-Infektionen trotz sinkender Fallzahlen weiterhin eine zentrale Rolle für die UV-Träger. Bei der BK 3101 entfielen bei der BGW im Jahr 2017 größere Anteile der anerkannten Fälle auf HCV-Infektionen, diese bildeten die größte Gruppe der BK mit neu bewilligten Renten (61). Zum wesentlichen Aufgabenbereich der gesetzlichen UV gehört im BK-Fall die Vorsorge vor Krankheitsfolgen sowie die Übernahme von Entschädigungsleistungen. Bei der CHC ist eine adäquate Behandlung mit dem Ziel der Virenfreiheit anzustreben, um das Fortschreiten der Erkrankung zu stoppen. Über Jahrzehnte ist die CHC als schwer therapierbare Infektion mit einer schweren Krankheitslast und hohen assoziierten Kosten verbunden gewesen.

Der wesentliche Inhalt der zweiten Publikation sind die Kosten der CHC als BK. Bis zur Zulassung der DAA wurden diese überwiegend von den kontinuierlich steigenden Ausgaben für Entschädigungsleistungen in Form von Renten bestimmt. Die Progredienz der chronischen Infektion führte im beobachteten Kollektiv zu Krankheitsfolgen mit entsprechender Anpassung der MdE und der Rentenleistungen. Für die Versicherten der UV ergeben sich Ansprüche auf eine Rentenleistung in Abhängigkeit vom Grad der MdE. Die Einschätzung der MdE als Grundlage einer Entschädigungsleistung für BK-Folgen orientiert sich in der Hauptsache an der entzündlichen Aktivität und am Grad der Fibrose beziehungsweise Zirrhose (49). Für die betroffenen Beschäftigten ging die CHC häufig mit erheblichen physischen und geistigen Beanspruchungen einher (10, 66). Nach erfolgreicher Therapie der HVC-Infektion fehlen die für die entzündliche Aktivität verantwortlichen RNA-Viren, fibrotische Umbauen bilden sich zurück, eine bestehende Zirrhose schreitet nicht weiter fort (47). Deshalb wird im Auftrag der UV nach einer erfolgreichen Therapie die MdE in einem Gutachten neu bewertet. Wie in der dritten Publikation berichtet, entfiel beziehungsweise reduzierte sich die MdE für 56 Versicherte nach erfolgreicher Therapie. Neben den medizinischen Kriterien müssen für die Einstufung der MdE im Gutachtenverfahren etwaige Beeinträchtigungen der beruflichen Situation durch BK-Folgen berücksichtigt werden (§ 56 Abs.

2 SGB VII (46)). Chronisch infizierten Beschäftigten blieben und bleiben unter Umständen Arbeitsbereiche verschlossen aufgrund des Schutzes Dritter (Patientenschutz), insbesondere betroffen von solchen Maßnahmen ist das operativ tätige medizinische Personal (57). Die Beeinträchtigung der beruflichen Situation bezieht sich gemäß Gesetzestext auf das gesamte Gebiet des Erwerbslebens. Die Berücksichtigung von Vorschädigungen bei der Bemessung der MdE nach einer effektiven Therapie schließt psychische Beeinträchtigungen als Folge der BK mit ein. Erst mit der Ent-wicklung der DAA wurden die Therapieoptionen für die Behandlung einer HCV-Infektion effektiver, durch orale interferonfreie Regime nebenwirkungsärmer und pangenotypisch einsetzbar.

Die Ergebnisse der DAA-Therapien bei BiG und deren potenzielle Auswirkungen auf die BK-Folgen sind Inhalt der dritten Publikation. Die untersuchten Ergebnisse der DAA-Therapien bestätigen die in der Literatur genannte ausgeprägte Effektivität dieser Medikamente. Das wichtigste Ergebnis dieser Studie ist der große therapeutische Erfolg (SVR12 94 %) in einem Versichertenkollektiv, das hauptsächlich therapieerfahren war und Leberschäden hatte. Als Prädiktor für eine statistisch signifikant geringere SVR-Rate erwies sich eine bereits bestehende Leberzirrhose (Zirrhose versus keine Zirrhose, 86 % versus 98 % SVR12-Raten, p = 0,006). Durch die verbesserte Prognose für die Heilung der CHC ist zukünftig mit geringeren manifesten Lebererkrankungen zu rechnen. Wie in der zweiten Publikation berichtet, machten in den Jahren 2000 bis 2014 60 % der aufsummierten Kosten allein die Rentenzahlungen aus. Kosten-Effektivitäts-Modellanalysen (35 Studien), die im Review von Nuno Solinis und Kollegen (41) analysiert wurden, zeigten, dass trotz der aktuell hohen Medikamentenpreise interferonfreie DAA-Therapien kosteneffektiver sind als frühere interferonhaltige Therapien, trotz der aktuell hohen Medikamentenpreise. Die Behandlung von Patienten in weniger schweren Krankheitsstadien mit einer DAA-Therapie verhindert bei Erfolg die Progredienz der Erkrankung. Es konnten bereits in den milden und gemäßigten Phasen der CHC erhebliche Kosten reduziert werden durch das Erreichen von SVR (67). Obwohl die Therapieerfolge überzeugend sind und in Deutschland jeder CHC-Erkrankte grundsätzlich Zugang zu einer DAA-Therapie hat, sind die Verschreibungszahlen bei den gesetzlich Versicherten insgesamt seit Ende 2015 rückläufig (24, 72). Als mögliche Gründe werden Unsicherheiten bezüglich der Leistungsgenehmigung sowie eine mögliche Überschätzung der Anzahl der diagnostizierten CHC-Erkrankten genannt. Eine Therapie setzt das Wissen um die Betroffenheit voraus.

Wissenschaftler gehen davon aus, dass die Dunkelziffer der Personen mit einer HCV-Infektion allein in Deutschland bei ca. 100.000 Personen liegt (75). Laut WHO haben weltweit weniger als 5 % der chronisch Hepatitis-Erkrankten (B und C) Kenntnis von ihrem Status (44). Über fehlende verbindliche Screening-Strategien für Risikogruppen wird international diskutiert (44, 72, 75). Deren Implementierung zur Identifizierung infizierter Personen und zur Unterbrechung von Infektionskanälen ist neben einer frühen effektiven Therapie eine wichtige Präventionsmaßnahme (75). Die HCV-Infektion ist weder impfpräventabel noch bietet eine bereits durchgemachte oder erfolgreich therapierte Infektion Schutz vor einer Neuinfektion (71, 76). Deshalb ist es notwendig, die regelmäßige Vorsorge bei Infektionsgefährdung entsprechend der ArbMedVV allen Beschäftigten anzubieten, um nach Kontakt, z. B. durch eine NSV, eine Neuinfektion auszuschließen. Die wichtigste Maßnahme zur Vermeidung einer beruflich erworbenen HCV-Infektion ist die Verhütung von NSV. Das Verwenden von stichsicheren Instrumenten (SSI) ist ein wichtiger Schritt. Allerdings ereignet sich ein Großteil der NSV bei der Entsorgung von Kanülen und anderen scharfen oder spitzen Instrumenten (51). Schulungen zum sicheren Umgang mit und zur Entsorgung von diesen Instrumenten sollten für alle Berufsgruppen regelmäßig angeboten werden. Aufgrund der hohen Dunkelziffer nicht gemeldeter NSV (7, 53) sollte der Umgang mit NSV ebenfalls thematisiert werden. Diese sollten dokumentiert und, einschließlich der wichtigsten Informationen zum Indexpatienten, als Arbeitsunfälle gemeldet werden. Die epidemiologische Erfassung und Auswertung können für die Entwicklung zielgerichteter Präventionsmaßnahmen von großem Nutzen sein.

Limitationen und Stärken

Die für die Metaanalyse vorgefundene Literatur bestand überwiegend aus Studien mit retrospektivem Design, in denen BiG häufig unabhängig vom Tätigkeitsprofil und unter Berücksichtigung uneinheitlicher Störfaktoren untersucht wurden. Viele der Kontrollen sind Blutspender, hierbei handelt es sich um eine selektive Klientel. Personen, die Blut spenden, legen möglicherweise ein anderes Gesundheitsverhalten an den Tag als die Allgemeinbevölkerung, Risikogruppen sind in der Regel nicht vertreten. Die Ergebnisse der Studien, die keine Kontrollgruppe untersuchen, sondern auf eine Untersuchung in der Allgemeinbevölkerung als Referenz hinweisen, müssen ebenfalls kritisch bewertet werden. Die BiG und die Kontrollgruppen sind möglicherweise nicht unter identischen Bedingungen untersucht worden. Die Qualität der eingesetzten Bestätigungstests in den Studien unterscheidet sich. Mögliche Gründe sind die Entwicklung besserer Nachweise, die Qualität der Durchführung sowie der Umstand, dass die Antigene der eingesetzten Such- und Bestätigungstests sich nicht grundlegend voneinander unterscheiden.

Die Variationen im Design bezüglich des untersuchten Beschäftigtenkollektivs und die fehlenden Kontrollen führten zu einem Mangel an Konsens in der Einschätzung des beruflichen Risikos für eine HCV-Infektion bei BiG. Dies ist das erste systematische Review, das unter Berücksichtigung der Studienqualität und von bestätigten serologischen HCV-Nachweisen eine quantitative Analyse der HCV-Prävalenz bei BiG im Vergleich zu nicht exponierten Kontrollen vornimmt. Die Umstände heute haben sich in Bezug auf die Falldefinition verändert. Für zukünftige Analysen sollten Studien berücksichtigt werden, die zusätzlich zu den reaktiven HCV-Nachweisen auch Viren-RNA-Nachweise durchführen und diese in einem Bestätigungstest kontrollieren.

Die Ergebnisse zur HCV-Infektion als BK basieren auf dem Datensatz der BGW und erfassen nur die BK-Meldungen der Beschäftigten aus nicht staatlichen Einrichtungen. Die Analysen basieren auf dem elektronisch erfassten Datensatz der BK-DOK. Für diese Registerdaten gelten die Einschränkungen, die für Sekundärdaten im Allgemeinen gelten. Es handelt sich um Verwaltungsdaten mit begrenzten soziodemografischen Merkmalen. Diese Daten weisen einen längsschnittlichen Verlauf auf und erlauben die Beobachtung der Inanspruchnahme von Versicherungsleistungen als relevante Outcomes über einen ausreichend langen Zeitraum. So können im Gegensatz zu Beobachtungen im Querschnittdesign Trends bei beruflich bedingten Erkrankungen dargestellt werden.

Bei der Analyse der Ergebnisse der DAA-Therapien bei BiG konnten die Angaben zu Koinfektionen aus dem Datensatz nicht valide ausgewertet werden, sie wurden nicht standardisiert abgefragt. Es ist allerdings von einer geringen Wahrscheinlichkeit einer Koinfektion auszugehen, da es sich im untersuchten Kollektiv um BiG handelt. Diese werden regelmäßig betriebsärztlich untersucht, was eine Kontrolle des HBV-Impfstatus einschließt. Drei Viertel der beobachteten Versicherten sind weiblich. Männer sind häufiger als Frauen von HCV-Infektionen sowie von einem chronischen Verlauf betroffen. Sie gehören häufiger Risikogruppen an, wie z.B. IVD, MSM, und sind öfter HIV-koinfiziert (44, 76). Zwischenergebnisse aus der GECCO-Studie bestätigen, dass Männer signifikant häufiger von einer HCV-HIV-Koinfektion betroffen sind als Frauen (27). In unserer Untersuchung deutet sich ebenfalls ein geschlechtsspezifischer Trend an, dieser sollte aufgrund der geringen Anzahl an Männern in der Stichprobe in zukünftigen Untersuchungen mit höheren Fallzahlen überprüft werden.

Um das Risiko für eine Hepatitis-B-Reaktivierung im Zusammenhang mit direkt wirkenden antiviralen Wirkstoffen zu minimieren, empfiehlt die Europäische Arzneimittel-Agentur (EMA) seit Dezember 2016 ein Hepatitis-B-Screening vor Beginn einer DAA-Behandlung. Die HBV-Reaktivierung wurde in Einzelfällen beobachtet und es wird vermutet, dass es sich um eine Folge der Reduktion der HCV-RNA-Viren handelt. Bei einer HCV-HBV-Koinfektion wird das HBV unterdrückt. Patienten, die sowohl HBV- als auch HCV-infiziert sind, müssen überwacht und gemäß den aktuellen Leitlinien behandelt werden (77).

Bei der global verbreiteten HCV-Infektion gibt es Erfolge bei den berufsspezifischen Präventionsmaßnahmen. Sowohl im amerikanischen als auch im europäischen Raum gibt es seit dem Jahr 2000 Richtlinien, um Expositionen mit infiziertem Blut durch NSV vorzubeugen (7, 78). Als Ergebnisse großer Public-Health-Kampagnen werden Rückgänge der Prävalenz in der Allgemeinbevölkerung in einigen Ländern beobachtet, wie z. B. in Ägypten, das zu den Hochprävalenzländern gehört (24). Obwohl sich ein Trendwechsel durch die Entwicklung der antiviralen Medikamente zur Behandlung der CHC-Infektionen abzeichnet, haben nicht alle Betroffenen Zugang zu den neuen effektiven Therapien. Bei der großen Mehrheit bleibt die Erkrankung unerkannt und unbehandelt. Der Zugang sowohl zur Diagnostik als auch zu den teuren DAA ist in vielen Ländern problematisch. Um möglichst allen CHC-Erkrankten eine verbesserte Therapieprognose zugänglich zu machen, wurde 2017 ein pangenotypisch antivirales Kombinationspräparat in die „Essential Medicines List" (EML) aufgenommen (1). Die WHO verfolgt durch ihre „Global Health Sector Strategy on Viral Hepatitis" aus dem Jahr 2016 das Ziel, die Virushepatitis (B und C) bis zum Jahr 2030 zu eliminieren. Dies soll unter anderem erreicht werden durch die Schaffung von Chancengleichheit beim Zugang zu Präventionsmaßnahmen und diagnostischen sowie therapeutischen Leistungen. Das Bundesministerium für Gesundheit und das Bundesministerium für wirtschaftliche Zusammenarbeit und Entwicklung knüpfen an die globale WHO-Strategie mit der „Strategie zur Eindämmung von HIV, HBV und HCV und anderen sexuell übertragbaren Infektionen (STI) bis 2030 – Bedarfsorientiert – Integriert – Sektorenübergreifend" aus dem Jahr 2016 an (24).

1.7 Fazit

Ein Trendwechsel zeichnet sich für die HCV als Infektionskrankheit seit der Entwicklung der antiviralen Medikamente ab. Die in dieser kumulativen Arbeit untersuchten Zusammenhänge helfen, das Risiko für eine berufsbedingte HCV-Infektion und deren Folgen sowohl für die BiG als auch für die UV einzuordnen und zu bewerten. Die Analyse der assoziierten Kosten der CHC und die zügige Untersuchung der Ergebnisse der DAA-Therapien bei den Beschäftigten bieten wichtige Erkenntnisse für den Umgang mit der HCV als BK.

Für die BiG bedeuten die verbesserten und effektiveren Therapiemöglichkeiten eine wesentlich günstigere Prognose insgesamt, vor allem beruflich. Mit den hohen Erfolgsraten der neuen Therapien, durchgeführt in einem frühen Krankheitsstadium, dürften langfristig progrediente Verläufe sowie Leberschädigungen und deren Folgen vermieden werden. Durch den Erhalt der Arbeitsfähigkeit ließen sich langfristig Kosteneinsparungen für die UV und für die sozialen Sicherungssysteme insgesamt erreichen. Allerdings benötigen wir langfristige Erfahrungen mit den DAA-Therapien, um die Ergebnisse valide interpretieren zu können.

Die hohen Erfolgsraten der HCV-Therapien ändern die Situation im BK-Geschehen. Eine aktuelle Fragestellung betrifft die individuelle Krankheitslast, die nach einer erfolgreichen Behandlung möglicherweise bei den Versicherten mit langer Krankheitsdauer bestehen bleibt. Vor allem die gerechte Bewertung der individuellen Krankheitslast nach Erreichen von SVR und die entsprechende Einstufung der MdE zeichnen sich als aktuelle Herausforderungen für die UV ab.

Diese Erkenntnisse lassen sich nicht aus den Routinedaten allein gewinnen. Hierfür sind empirische Untersuchungen notwendig. Aktuell werden die Daten einer Befragung von BiG mit einer CHC als BK im Rahmen einer Prä-Post-Studie zur Wirksamkeit der angebotenen Heilbehandlung ausgewertet. Die Ergebnisse zur Arbeitsfähigkeit, zur gesundheitsbezogenen Lebensqualität und zur Angst- und Depressionssymptomatik sollen in nachhaltige Konzepte für die Versorgung der Versicherten durch die UV einfließen.

Eine zweite aktuelle Fragestellung soll anhand einer Kosten-Effektivitäts-Analyse untersucht werden. Die Entwicklung der Kosten der beruflichen HCV-Infektion, insbesondere der Trend bei den Rentenleistungen vor und nach Einführung der DAA, soll anhand der Daten einer UV retrospektiv und anhand von Modellen prospektiv gesundheitsökonomisch betrachtet werden.

Über die „Vision null Infektionen" wird international und national, auch innerhalb der UV, diskutiert. Bei der HCV als BK sind in Deutschland die Voraussetzungen dafür aktuell besser denn je. Mit den DAA stehen effiziente und gut verträgliche Therapien allen BiG zur Verfügung, für die Prophylaxe ist der Zugang und der geschulte Umgang mit SSI für alle betroffenen Berufe im Gesundheitsdienst anzustreben. Hier besteht noch Handlungsbedarf. NSV sollten regelmäßig erfasst und ausgewertet werden, das Risiko einer berufsbedingten HCV-Infektion und die daraus resultierenden Folgen sollte auch zukünftig wissenschaftlich betrachtet werden.

1.8 Literaturverzeichnis

1. **WHO.** Global hepatitis report 2017 [Internet]. 2017 [zitiert am 27.11.2018]. URL: http://www.who.int/iris/handle/10665/255016

2. **Blachier M, Leleu H, Peck-Radosavljevic M, Valla DC, Roudot-Thoraval F.** The burden of liver disease in Europe: a review of available epidemiological data. J Hepatol. 2013;58(3):593-608.

3. **Gomaa AI, Waked I.** Recent advances in multidisciplinary management of hepatocellular carcinoma. World J Hepatol. 2015;7(4):673-87.

4. **Russmann S, Dowlatshahi EA, Printzen G, Habicht S, Reichen J, Zimmermann H.** Prevalence and associated factors of viral hepatitis and transferrin elevations in 5036 patients admitted to the emergency room of a Swiss university hospital: cross-sectional study. BMC Gastroenterol. 2007;7:5.

5. **Wicker S, Rabenau HF, Groneberg DA, Gottschalk R.** Arbeitsbedingte Infektionen bei Mitarbeitern des Gesundheitswesens: Blutübertragbare Erkrankungen. Zbl. Arbeitsmed. 2009;59(5):138-50.

6. **Deuffic-Burban S, Delarocque-Astagneau E, Abiteboul D, Bouvet E, Yazdanpanah Y.** Blood-borne viruses in health care workers: prevention and management. J Clin Virol. 2011;52(1):4-10.

7. **Elseviers MM, Arias-Guillen M, Gorke A, Arens HJ.** Sharps injuries amongst healthcare workers: review of incidence, transmissions and costs. J Ren Care. 2014;40(3):150-6.

8. **Remé T.** Arbeitsmedizinische Grundlagen für die Konkretisierung von Beweiserleichterungen im Berufskrankheitenfeststellungsverfahren - Fallgruppen und Einzelfallermittlungen. In: Selmair H, Manns MP, Hrsg. Virushepatitis als Berufskrankheit: Ein Leitfaden zur Begutachtung. 3. Aufl. Landsberg: ecomed 2007; 227-38.

9. **Sozialgesetzbuch (SGB VII)** – Siebtes Buch – Gesetzliche Unfallversicherung (Zuletzt geändert durch Art. 4 G v. 17.7.2017 I 2575) § 9 SGB VII Berufskrankheit [Internet]. 2018 [zitiert am 7.12.2018]. URL: https://www.sozialgesetzbuch-sgb.de/sgbvii/9.html.

10. **Quelhas R, Lopes A.** Psychiatric problems in patients infected with hepatitis C before and during antiviral treatment with interferon-alpha: a review. J Psychiatr Pract. 2009;15(4):262-81.

11. **Lim JK.** Natural history of hepatitis C infection: a concise review. Yale J Biol Med. 2001;74(4):229-37.

12. **Gerlach JT, Diepolder HM, Jung MC, Grüner NH, Zachoval R, Schirren CA, et al.** Akute Hepatitis C. Dtsch Ärztebl. 1999;96(48):A-3103-6.

13. **Polywka S.** Diagnostische Verfahren bei der Hepatitis C und ihre Zuverlässigkeit. In: Selmair H, Manns MP, Hrsg. Virushepatitis als Berufskrankheit: Ein Leitfaden zur Begutachtung. Landsberg: ecomed; 2007: 44-56.

14. **Bartenschlager R.** Hepatitis-C-Virus. In: Doerr HW, Gerlich WH, Hrsg. Medizinische Virologie Grundlagen, Diagnostik, Prävention und Therapie viraler Erkrankungen. 2. Aufl. Stuttgart: Georg Thieme Verlag; 2010: 402-8.

15. **Gerold G, Pietschmann T.** The HCV life cycle: in vitro tissue culture systems and therapeutic targets. Dig Dis. 2014;32(5):525-37.

16. **Zachoval R, Jung MC.** Aktuelle Therapieoptionen bei chronischer Hepatitis C [Chronic Hepatitis C - Therapeutic Options in 2016]. MMW Fortschr Med. 2016;158 Suppl 1:54-7.

17. **Isken O, Langerwisch U, Jirasko V, Rehders D, Redecke L, Ramanathan H, Lindenbach BD, Bartenschlager R, Tautz N.** A conserved NS3 surface patch orchestrates NS2 protease stimulation, NS5A hyperphosphorylation and HCV genome replication. PLoS Pathog. 2015;11(3):e1004736.

18. **Smith DB, Bukh J, Kuiken C, Muerhoff AS, Rice CM, Stapleton JT, Simmonds P.** Expanded classification of hepatitis C virus into 7 genotypes and 67 subtypes: updated criteria and genotype assignment web resource. Hepatology (Baltimore, Md). 2014;59(1):318-27.

19. **Sarrazin C, Zimmermann T, Berg T, Neumann UP, Schirmacher P, Schmidt H, Spengler U, Timm J, Wedemeyer H, Wirth S, Zeuzem S.** Deutsche Gesellschaft für Gastroenterologie, Verdauungs-und Stoffwechselkrankheiten, Deutsche Gesellschaft für Pathologie e.V., Deutsche Leberstiftung, Gesellschaft für Virologie e.V., Gesellschaft für Padiatrische Gastroenterologie und Ernährung, Österreichische Gesellschaft für Gastroenterologie und Hepatologie, Schweizerische Gesellschaft für Gastroenterologie, Deutsche Transplantationsgesellschaft e. V., Deutsche Leberhilfe e. V., Deutsche Gesellschaft für Infektiologie e. V., Deutsche Gesell-schaft für Suchtmedizin e. V., Deutsche Aids-Gesellschaft e. V., Deutsche Arbeitsgemeinschaft niedergelassener Ärzte für die Versorgung HIV-Infizierter, Robert Koch-Institut. S3-Leitlinie „Prophylaxe, Diagnostik und Therapie der Hepatitis-C-Virus (HCV)-Infektion". Z Gastroenterol. 2018;56(7):756-838.

20. **Sarrazin C, Berg T, Ross RS, Schirmacher P, Wedemeyer H, Neumann U, Schmidt HH, Spengler U, Wirth S, Kessler HH, Peck-Radosavljevic M, Ferenci P, Vogel W, Moradpour D, Heim M, Cornberg M, Protzer U, Manns MP, Fleig WE, Dollinger MM, Zeuzem S.** Update der S 3-Leitlinie Prophylaxe, Diagnostik und Therapie der Hepatitis-C-Virus(HCV)-Infektion, AWMF-Register-Nr.: 021/021 [Prophylaxis, diagnosis and therapy of hepatitis C virus (HCV) infection: the German guidelines on the management of HCV infection]. Z Gastroenterol. 2010;48(2):289-351.

21. **RKI.** RKI-Ratgeber Hepatitis C. Epid Bull. 2018;2018(31):299-307.

22. **Poethko-Muller C, Zimmermann R, Hamouda O, Faber M, Stark K, Ross RS, Thamm M.** Die Seroepidemiologie der hepatitis A, B und C in Deutschland: Ergebnisse der Studie zur Gesundheit Erwachsener in Deutschland (DEGS1) [Epidemiology of hepatitis A, B, and C among adults in Germany: results of the German Health Interview and Examination Survey for Adults (DEGS1)]. Bundesgesundheitsblatt, Gesundheitsforschung, Gesundheitsschutz. 2013;56(5-6):707-15.

23. **Just H-M.** Rechtliche Grundlagen und hygienerelevante Gesetzgebung. In: Schulz-Stübner S, Hrsg. Repetitorium Krankenhaushygiene und hygienebeauftragter Arzt. Berlin, Heidelberg: Springer Berlin Heidelberg; 2013: 1-32.

24. **Zimmermann R, Meurs L, Schmidt D, Kollan C, Dudareva S, Bremer V.** Hepatitis C im Jahr 2017. Zur Situation bei wichtigen Infektionskrankheiten in Deutschland. Epid Bull. 2018;2018(29):271-84.

25. **Askarian M, Yadollahi M, Kuochak F, Danaei M, Vakili V, Momeni M.** Precautions for health care workers to avoid hepatitis B and C virus infection. Int J Occup Environ Med. 2011;2(4):191-8.

26. **Zimmermann R, Seidel J, Simeonova Y, Schmidt D, Dudareva-Vizule S, Bremer V.** Hepatitis C im Jahr 2016. Zur Situation bei wichtigen Infektionskrankheiten in Deutschland. Epid Bull. 2017;2017(30):279-90.

27. **Ingiliz P, Christensen S, Kimhofer T, Hueppe D, Lutz T, Schewe K, et al.** Sofosbuvir and Ledipasvir for 8 Weeks for the Treatment of Chronic Hepatitis C Virus (HCV) Infection in HCV-Monoinfected and HIV-HCV-Coinfected Individuals: Results From the German Hepatitis C Cohort (GECCO-01). Clin. Infect. Dis. 2016;63(10):1320-4.

28. **Benova L, Mohamoud YA, Calvert C, Abu-Raddad LJ.** Vertical transmission of hepatitis C virus: systematic review and meta-analysis. Clin. Infect. Dis. 2014;59(6):765-73.

29. **Yeung CY, Lee HC, Chan WT, Jiang CB, Chang SW, Chuang CK.** Vertical transmission of hepatitis C virus: Current knowledge and perspectives. World J Hepatol. 2014;6(9):643-51.

30. **Holz L, Rehermann B.** T cell responses in hepatitis C virus infection: historical overview and goals for future research. Antiviral Res. 2015;114:96-105.

31. **Younossi ZM, Singer ME, Mir HM, Henry L, Hunt S.** Impact of interferon free regimens on clinical and cost outcomes for chronic hepatitis C genotype 1 patients. J Hepatol. 2014;60(3):530-7.

32. **Diepolder HM, Zachoval R, Hoffmann RM, Jung MC, Gerlach T, Pape GR.** The role of hepatitis C virus specific CD4+ T lymphocytes in acute and chronic hepatitis C. J Mol Med (Berl). 1996;74(10):583-8.

33. **Kraus MR, Wilms K.** Interferon-αWirkung, Indikationen, Therapieüberwachung und Nebenwirkungen. Internist (Berl). 2000;41(12):1399-406.

34. **Heintges TE, A.; Wenning, M.; Häussinger, D.** Pegyliertes (PEG-) Interferon : Eine neue Therapieoption bei chronischer Hepatitis C. Dtsch Ärztebl Int. 2001;98(4):182-.

35. **Kohli A, Shaffer A, Sherman A, Kottilil S.** Treatment of hepatitis C: a systematic review. JAMA. 2014;312(6):631-40.

36. **Lok AS, Gardiner DF, Lawitz E, Martorell C, Everson GT, Ghalib R, Reindollar R, Rustgi V, McPhee F, Wind-Rotolo M, Persson A, Zhu K, Dimitrova DI, Eley T, Guo T, Grasela DM, Pasquinelli C.** Preliminary study of two antiviral agents for hepatitis C genotype 1. N Engl J Med. 2012;366(3):216-24.

37. **Lubel J, Strasser S, Stuart KA, Dore G, Thompson A, Pianko S, Bollipo S, Mitchell JL, Fragomeli V, Jones T, Chivers S, Gow P, Iser D, Levy M, Tse E, Gazzola A, Cheng W, Nazareth S, Galhenage S, Wade A, Weltman M, Wigg A, MacQuillan G, Sasadeusz J, George J, Zekry A, Roberts SK.** Australian Liver Association Clinical Research Network. Real-world efficacy and safety of ritonavir-boosted paritaprevir, ombitasvir, dasabuvir +/- ribavirin for hepatitis C genotype 1 – final results of the REV1TAL study. Antivir Ther. 2017;22(8):699-710.

38. **Surjadi M.** Chronic Hepatitis C Screening, Evaluation, and Treatment Update in the Age of Direct-Acting Antivirals. Workplace Health Saf. 2018;66(6):302-9.

39. **Sarrazin C, Zeuzem S.** Leitliniengerechte Therapie der Hepatitis C. Die Eradikation von HCV als Ziel [Current Guidelines for treatment of hepatitis C. The eradication of HCV as a goal]. Pharm Unserer Zeit. 2011;40(1):52-9.

40. **Gonzalez-Grande R, Jimenez-Perez M, Gonzalez Arjona C, Mostazo Torres J.** New approaches in the treatment of hepatitis C. World J Gastroenterol. 2016;22(4):1421-32.

41. **Nuno Solinis R, Arratibel Ugarte P, Rojo A, Sanchez Gonzalez Y.** Value of Treating All Stages of Chronic Hepatitis C: A Comprehensive Review of Clinical and Economic Evidence. Infect Dis Ther. 2016;5(4):491-508.

42. **Stahmeyer JT, Krauth C, Bert F, Pfeiffer-Vornkahl H, Alshuth U, Huppe D, Mauss S, Rossol S.** Costs and outcomes of treating chronic hepatitis C patients in routine care – results from a nationwide multicenter trial. J Viral Hepat. 2016;23(2):105-15.

43. **Tada T, Kumada T, Toyoda H, Kiriyama S, Tanikawa M, Hisanaga Y, Kanamori A, Kitabatake S, Yama T, Tanaka J.** Viral eradication reduces all-cause mortality in patients with chronic hepatitis C virus infection: a propensity score analysis. Liver Int. 2016;36(6):817-26.

44. **WHO.** Global Health Sector Strategy On Viral Hepatitis 2016–2021 Towards Ending Viral Hepatitis [Internet] 2016 [zitiert am 27.11.2018]. URL: http://www.who.int/hepatitis/strategy2016-2021/ghss-hep/en/

45. **Auhuber TC, Reimertz C, Müller WD, Hoffmann R.** Neuausrichtung der Heilverfahren der Gesetzlichen Unfallversicherung. Orthopädie und Unfallchirurgie up2date. 2015;10(01):51-69.

46. **Sozialgesetzbuch (SGB VII)** – Siebtes Buch – Gesetzliche Unfallversicherung (Zuletzt geändert durch Art. 4 G v. 17.7.2017 I 2575) § 56 SGB VII Voraussetzungen und Höhe des Rentenanspruchs [Internet] 2018 [zitiert am 27.11.2018]. URL: https://www.sozialgesetzbuch-sgb.de/sgbvii/56html.

47. **Nienhaus A.** Hepatitis-C-Virus-Infektionen im Gesundheitswesen. Therapie der akuten und chronischen Infektion. ASU Arbeitsmed Sozialmed Umweltmed. 2018;53(1):13-5.

48. **Mehrtens G, Valentin H, Schönberger A.** Arbeitsunfall und Berufskrankheit. Rechtliche und medizinische Grundlagen für Gutachter, Sozialverwaltung, Berater und Gerichte. 9. Aufl., Berlin: Erich Schmidt Verlag; 2017.

49. **Selmair H, Ohlen J, Korb G, Hopf U, Schneider W, Brandenburg S.** Zur gutachterlichen Bewertung (MdE) der chronischen Virushepatitis B und C und deren Folgezustände in der gesetzlichen Unfallversicherung. In: Selmair H, Manns MP, Eds. Virushepatitis als Berufskrankheit: Ein Leitfaden zur Begutachtung. Landesberg: ecomed MEDIZIN; 2007: 247-57.

50. **Wendeler D, Dulon M, Nienhaus A.** Unfälle und Berufskrankheiten im Jahr 2016 bei der Berufsgenossenschaft für Gesundheitsdienst und Wohlfahrtspflege. In: Nienhaus A, Eds. RiRe – Risiken und Ressourcen in Gesundheitsdienst und Wohlfahrtspflege. 3. Aufl. Landesberg: ecomed; 2018: 9-30.

51. **Dulon M, Lisiak B, Wendeler D, Nienhaus A.** Unfallmeldungen zu Nadelstichverletzungen bei Beschäftigten in Krankenhausern, Arztpraxen und Pflegeeinrichtungen. [Workers' Compensation Claims for Needlestick Injuries Among Healthcare Personnel in Hospitals, Doctor's Surgeries and Nursing Institutions]. Gesundheitswesen. 2018;80(2):176-82.

52. **Nienhaus A, Kesavachandran C, Wendeler D, Haamann F, Dulon M.** Infectious diseases in healthcare workers - an analysis of the standardised data set of a German compensation board. J Occup Med Toxicol. 2012;7(1):8.

53. **Himmelreich H, Rabenau HF, Rindermann M, Stephan C, Bickel M, Marzi I, Wicker S.** The management of needlestick injuries. Dtsch Ärztebl Int. 2013;110(5):61-7.

54. **Kubitschke A, Bahr MJ, Aslan N, Bader C, Tillmann HL, Sarrazin C, Greten T, Wiegand J, Manns MP, Wedemeyer H.** Induction of hepatitis C virus (HCV)-specific T cells by needle stick injury in the absence of HCV-viraemia. Eur J Clin Invest. 2007;37(1):54-64.

55. **Tomkins SE, Elford J, Nichols T, Aston J, Cliffe SJ, Roy K, et al.** Occupational transmission of hepatitis C in healthcare workers and factors associated with seroconversion: UK surveillance data. J Viral Hepat. 2012;19(3):199-204.

56. **Yazdanpanah Y, De Carli G, Migueres B, Lot F, Campins M, Colombo C, Thomas T, Deuffic-Burban S, Prevot MH, Domart M, Tarantola A, Abiteboul D, Deny P, Pol S, Desenclos JC, Puro V, Bouvet E.** Risk factors for hepatitis C virus transmission to health care workers after occupational exposure: a European case-control study. Clinical infectious diseases: Open Forum Infect Dis. 2005;41(10):1423-30.

57. **Hofmann F.** Zur nosokomialen Übertragung von Hepatitis-B- und Hepatitis-C-Viren durch Beschäftigte im Gesundheitsdienst. Arbeitsmed Sozialmed Umweltmed. 2015;50(6):439-45.

58. **BMJV.** Biostoffverordnung vom 15. Juli 2013 (BGBl. I S. 2514), die zuletzt durch Artikel 146 des Gesetzes vom 29. März 2017 (BGBl. I S. 626) geändert worden ist. BGBl [Inernet]. 2013. [zitiert am 27.11.2018]. URL: https://www.gesetze-im-internet.de/biostoffv_2013/BJNR251410013.html

59. **Ausschuss für Biologische Arbeitsstoffe (ABAS) AfBA.** Technische Regeln für Biologische Arbeitsstoffe: Biologische Arbeitsstoffe im Gesundheitswesen und in der Wohlfahrtspflege – TRBA 250 4. Änderung vom 2.5.2018 GMBI. 2014(10-11):206.

60. **Stranzinger JW, Wunderle W, Dulon M, Nienhaus A, Kaise B, Steinmann J, Jung S, Polywka, S.** Konsenspapier zur Nachsorge von Stich- und Schnittverletzungen mit infektiösen Material – Gemeinsame Empfehlungen der Unfallkassen Baden-Würtenberg, Berlin, Nord, Nordrhein-Westfalen und der Berufsgenossenschaft für Gesundheitsdienst und Wohlfahrtspflege. ASU Arbeitsmed Sozialmed Praventivmed. 2018;53:248-55.

61. **Dulon M, Wendeler D, Nienhaus A.** Berufsbedingte Infektionskrankheiten bei Beschäftigten im Gesundheitsdienst 2017: Routinedaten der Berufsgenossenschaft für Gesundheitsdienst und Wohlfahrtspflege 2018. Zbl Arbeitsmed. 2018. DOI/10.1007/s40664-018-0307-4

62. **Gordon SC, Pockros PJ, Terrault NA, Hoop RS, Buikema A, Nerenz D, Hamzeh FM.** Impact of disease severity on healthcare costs in patients with chronic hepatitis C (CHC) virus infection. Hepatology (Baltimore, Md). 2012;56(5):1651-60.

63. **Tillmann HL, Wiese M, Braun Y, Wiegand J, Tenckhoff S, Mossner J, Manns M.P, Weissenborn, K.** Quality of life in patients with various liver diseases: patients with HCV show greater mental impairment, while patients with PBC have greater physical impairment. J Viral Hepat. 2011;18(4):252-61.

64. **Hilsabeck RC, Hassanein TI, Carlson MD, Ziegler EA, Perry W.** Cognitive functioning and psychiatric symptomatology in patients with chronic hepatitis C. Journal of the International Neuropsychological Society: J Int Neuropsychol Soc. 2003;9(6):847-54.

65. **Stahmeyer JT, Rossol S, Bert F, Abdelfattah M, Wiebner B, Wedemeyer H, et al.** Die Kosten der Versorgung von Hepatitis C Patienten in Deutschland. Gesundheitswesen. 2013;75(08/09):A274.

66. **Sarrazin C BT, Buggisch P, Dollinger MM, Hinrichsen H, Hofer H et al.** Aktuelle Empfehlung zur Therapie der chronischen Hepatitis C [S3 guideline hepatitis C addendum]. Z Gastroenterol. 2015;53:320–34.

67. **Nevens F, Colle I, Michielsen P, Robaeys G, Moreno C, Caekelbergh K, et al.** Resource use and cost of hepatitis C-related care. Eur J Gastroenterol Hepatol. 2012;24(10):1191-8.

68. **Westbrook RH, Dusheiko G.** Natural history of hepatitis C. J. Hepatol. 2014;61(1 Suppl):S58-68.

69. **Fagiuoli S, Ravasio R, Lucà MG, Baldan A, Pecere S, Vitale A, et al.** Management of hepatitis C infection before and after liver transplantation. World J Gastroenterol. 2015;21(15):4447-56.

70. **Westermann C, Dulon M, Wendeler D, Nienhaus A.** Hepatitis C among healthcare personnel: secondary data analyses of costs and trends for hepatitis C infections with occupational causes. J Occup Med Toxicol. 2016;11:52.

71. **Zeuzem S.** Treatment Options in Hepatitis C. Dtsch Arztebl Int. 2017;114(1-02):11-21.

72. **Zimmermann R, Kollan C, Ingiliz P, Mauss S, Schmidt D, Bremer V.** Real-world treatment for chronic hepatitis C infection in Germany: Analyses from drug prescription data, 2010–2015. J. Hepatol. 2017;67(1):15-22.

73. **Schäfer M, Schwaiger M.** Interferon-α-assoziierte psychische Nebenwirkungen. Häufigkeit, Ursachen und Therapie [Incidence, pathoetiology and treatment of interferon-α induced neuro-psychiatric side effects]. Fortschr Neurol Psychiatr. 2003;71(09):469-76.

74. **Slim J, Afridi MS.** Managing adverse effects of interferon-alfa and ribavirin in combination therapy for HCV. Infect Dis Clin North Am. 2012;26(4):917-29.

75. **Warpakowski A.** Hepatitis C: Elimination in Europa möglich. Dtsch Ärztebl Int. 2016; 113(21):20.

76. **Webster DP, Klenerman P, Dusheiko GM.** Hepatitis C. Lancet. 2015;385(9973):1124-35.

77. **Bundesinstitut für Arzneimittel und Medizinprodukte.** Risikobewertungsverfahren. Direkt antiviral wirkende Arzneimittel zur Hepatitis-C-Behandlung: Mögliche Hepatitis-B Reaktivierung [Internet]. 2017 [zitiert am 22.10.2018]. URL: https://www.bfarm.de/SharedDocs/Risikoinformationen/Pharmakovigilanz/DE/RV_STP/a-f/daclastavir.html

78. **Phillips EK, Conaway MR, Jagger JC.** Percutaneous injuries before and after the Needlestick ‹Safety and Prevention Act. New Engl J Med. 2012;366(7):670-1.

2 Publikationen

Publikation 1

The prevalence of hepatitis C among healthcare workers: a systematic review and meta-analysis

Prävalenz der Hepatitis C bei Beschäftigten im Gesundheitswesen im Vergleich zur Allgemeinbevölkerung – Metaanalyse

Publikation 2

Hepatitis C among healthcare personnel: secondary data analyses of costs and trends for hepatitis C infections with occupational causes

Hepatitis C bei Beschäftigten im Gesundheitswesen: Sekundärdatenanalyse über Kosten und Trends für beruflich bedingte Hepatitis-C-Infektionen

Publikation 3

Hepatitis C in healthcare personnel: secondary data analysis of therapies with direct-acting antiviral agents

Hepatitis C bei Beschäftigten im Gesundheitswesen: Sekundärdatenanalyse zu den Therapien mit direkt antiviral wirksamen Medikamenten

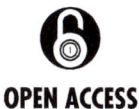

The prevalence of hepatitis C among healthcare workers: a systematic review and meta-analysis

Claudia Westermann,[1] Claudia Peters,[1] Birgitte Lisiak,[2] Monica Lamberti,[3] Albert Nienhaus[1,2]

▶ Additional material is published online only. To view please visit the journal online (http://dx.doi.org/10.1136/oemed-2015-102879).

[1]University Medical Center Hamburg-Eppendorf, Institute for Health Services Research in Dermatology and Nursing, Hamburg, Germany
[2]Institution for Statutory Accident Insurance and Prevention in Health and Welfare Services, Hamburg, Germany
[3]Department of Biochemistry, Biophysics and General Pathology, Second University of Naples, Naples, Italy

Correspondence to
Claudia Westermann, University Medical Center Hamburg-Eppendorf, Institute for Health Services Research in Dermatology and Nursing, Martinistrasse 52, Hamburg 20246, Germany; c.westermann@uke.de

Received 10 February 2015
Revised 5 August 2015
Accepted 30 August 2015
Published Online First 5 October 2015

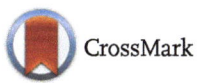

To cite: Westermann C, Peters C, Lisiak B, et al. Occup Environ Med 2015;**72**:880–888.

ABSTRACT
The aim of this study was to estimate the prevalence of viral hepatitis C (HCV) infection among healthcare workers (HCWs) compared to the general population. A systematic search for the years 1989–2014 was conducted in the Medline, Embase and Cochrane databases. Studies on hepatitis C in HCWs were included if they incorporated either a control group or reference data for the general population. The study quality was classified as high, moderate or low. Pooled effect estimates were calculated to determine the odds of occupational infection. Heterogeneity between studies was analysed using the χ^2 test ($p<0.10$) and quantified using the I^2 test. 57 studies met our criteria for inclusion and 44 were included in the meta-analysis. Analysis of high and moderate quality studies showed a significantly increased OR for HCV infection in HCWs relative to control populations, with a value of 1.6 (95% CI 1.03 to 2.42). Stratification by study region gave an OR of 2.1 in low prevalence countries; while stratification by occupational groups gave an increased prevalence for medical (OR 2.2) and for laboratory staff (OR 2.2). The OR for professionals at high risk of blood contact was 2.7. The pooled analysis indicates that the prevalence of infection is significantly higher in HCWs than in the general population. The highest prevalence was observed among medical and laboratory staff. Prospective studies that focus on HCW-specific activity and personal risk factors for HCV infection are needed.

INTRODUCTION
Viral hepatitis C (HCV) infection is caused by blood contact and is a public health problem throughout the world. Its clinical course may be severe and can lead to work disability or to death. Considerable costs are incurred for prophylactic and treatment measures and result from the chronic clinical progress of the disease, loss of working hours and premature death. According to the WHO, approximately 150 million people in the world are chronically infected with HCV, and hepatitis C is the cause of 350 000 deaths annually.[1] HCV is mainly transmitted by contact with infected blood due to injuries to the skin or mucous membranes.[2] Acute infection is often asymptomatic and therefore frequently overlooked. In up to 80% of patients, the clinical course is chronic, leading to an increased risk of developing hepatic cirrhosis or hepatic cell carcinoma.[3] Risk factors for HCV infection include intravenous drug consumption, injury-prone sex (men with men) and blood transfusions before the introduction of diagnostic testing. There is no vaccine or postexposure prophylaxis for HCV infection.

Healthcare workers (HCWs) have contact with infected patients and their body fluids. A particularly important factor is repeated performance of exposure prone procedures (EPPs) that may cause injuries to employees.[4] Injuries to medical and health staff from sharp or pointed objects are among the most frequently reported occupational accidents in healthcare.[5] The results of epidemiological studies indicate that approximately 80% of HCWs have been affected by needlestick injuries (NSI).[6] Many such injuries go unreported.[6–8] The risk of seroconversion after an injury depends on factors including the type of injury (deep cuts or pricks), the quantity of infectious material transferred, the virus load in the index patient and possibly genetic factors in the injured person.[8–10]

The probability of HCV seroconversion after a NSI in Europe has been estimated as 0.42%.[6] [8] Although HCV infection as an occupational disease is statistically rare, the consequences for the HCW and the health system are considerable.[7] [11] [12] In 2012, 79 HCV infections were reported to the German Institution for Statutory Accident Insurance and Prevention in Health and Welfare Services, and 47 infections were recognised as occupational diseases.[13] Numerous studies have investigated the prevalence of HCV in HCWs, but the results have been inconsistent. The objective of the present study is to estimate the prevalence of HCV infection among HCWs compared to the general population. Which professionals are particularly affected by infection?

METHODS
This study is reported in line with the Proposal for Reporting of Meta-analyses of Observational Studies (MOOSE).[14]

Search strategy and screening
A systematic literature search was performed in the Medline, Embase and Cochrane databases for the period from 1989 to 2014. This included all prevalence and incidence studies on hepatitis C in HCWs with either a control group or reference data on the general population. The Embase search was performed using the following search terms: ((((('hepatitis C') AND 'occupational exposure') AND 'healthcare worker') AND prevalence) OR incidence)—with and without truncation (see online supplementary file). The search strategy was adapted for the other databases. Additionally, we searched reference lists of the chosen studies and prior reviews. Where it was not possible to make a decision on a study's inclusion or exclusion based on the abstract, the full text of the study was

BMJ

examined. The studies were screened and their quality was assessed by two reviewers working independently and using pre-defined checklists. Disagreements were resolved by consensus.

Studies meeting the following criteria were considered for inclusion:

▶ Population: HCWs in direct contact with patients or blood
▶ Exposure: Study examines occupational exposure
▶ Control: Control group/reference data for general population from other publications
▶ Outcome: Serological test for HCV
▶ Design: Prevalence and incidence studies
▶ Languages: German, English, French, Spanish, Portuguese, Italian.

The following criteria led to exclusion from this study:

▶ Population: HCWs without direct contact with patients or blood
▶ Exposure: No occupational exposure
▶ Control: No control group; reference data for the general population not taken from other publications
▶ Outcome: No serological test for HCV
▶ Design: Case reports, surveillance data.

In studies with several control groups, the ones selected were those that best reflected the general population. Studies that examined HCWs without a control group were only included when the results were compared with a population-based study performed within a period of 2 years before or after the actual investigation and in a comparable study region.

In this report, 'healthcare worker' (HCW) is defined as any person (eg, an employee or student) whose activities involve contact with patients or with blood or other body fluids from patients in a healthcare setting.[15]

Study quality

In accordance with the literature, we developed an instrument to assess the methodological quality of the observational studies included.[16–20] Scores were awarded on the basis of the criteria below. A total of nine scores was possible (table 1).

Quality of the laboratory test: Anti-HCV detection depends on the type of test used, and tests differ in quality (product and procedure). In order to standardise the quality assessment, we evaluated the presence of a confirmatory test, but not its quality or procedure. It was not possible to evaluate this in the primary studies, due to missing data.

Statistical analysis

For the meta-analysis, data were extracted from the studies using a standardised documentation form. The parameters were

Table 1 Checklist for quality assessment

Item	Criterion	Content	Score
1	Aim	A clearly stated aim	1
2	Sample size	>50 persons	1
3	Response rate	>50%	1
4	Length of employment	Information is available	1
5	Control group	A control group was tested	1
6	Confounder	Adjusted for potential confounders	1
7	Limitations	Were discussed	1
8	Laboratory tests	Performance of anti-HCV test or PCR test	1
		Performance of confirmatory test	1

8–9 scores=high; 5–7 scores=moderate; ≤4 scores=low.
HCV, viral hepatitis C.

the number of employees examined and the proportion of employees tested as serologically positive. Prevalence ratios (ORs) were calculated as effect estimates using the Mantel-Haenszel method for dichotomous outcomes. The 95% CIs were generated. Additional analyses were performed after stratification by type of controls, study region, publication period, gender and professional group. Meta-analyses were carried out using Review Manager 5.2.

In accordance with the criteria of Trevisan *et al*,[50] a pooled analysis was performed for professionals exposed to a high risk of blood contact from EPPs. This analysis included the following professions/working areas: surgeons, midwives, microbiologists, pathologists, blood bank and dialysis staff.

Stratification by study region was performed on the basis of national prevalence rates. Based on the publications of Te and Jensen,[3] Hahne *et al*[21] and Mohd Hanafiah *et al*,[22] pooled effect estimates were calculated for low prevalence countries taking into account countries of north-west Europe and the USA. Studies from Japan were analysed separately as there have been reports that the rate of seroconversion is higher in Japan than in Europe.[8]

Studies that observed no HCV infection in either group were excluded from the meta-analysis as no information about the relative probability of the event could be derived.[18]

Heterogeneity and sensitivity analysis

The presence of heterogeneity was tested using the χ^2 test, taking $p<0.10$ as the level of significance. An I^2 test was performed to quantify the diversity between studies. If there was no evidence of heterogeneity, we used a variance approach with a fixed effect model.[18] In cases of statistically significant heterogeneity (χ^2 p value <0.10) and $I^2>50\%$, the pooled effect estimate was determined using the random effect model. To identify sources of variation, further stratification was performed relative to study quality and to performance of confirmatory tests. In addition, for the sensitivity analyses, the stability of the pooled estimate with respect to each study was investigated by excluding individual studies from the analysis.

Publication bias

Possible publication bias was visualised with a funnel plot. In addition, the probability of publication bias was tested using Egger's linear regression in SPSS V.20.[23] The level of significance for asymmetry was taken as $p<0.1$. The calculated intercept is given with a 90% confidence range.

RESULTS

A total of 3016 publications were identified in the databases and 41 by manual search. After checking for duplicates, the titles and abstracts of 954 studies were screened, leading to the exclusion of 801 studies. The full texts of 153 studies were scrutinised and 57 studies were included in the systematic review. This selection process is given in figure 1.

Table 2 gives an overview of the studies included. A total of 27 studies from Europe were included, along with 13 from Asia, eight from Africa, seven from North America and two from South America. In most studies, HCWs were examined within the inter-professional framework. In five studies, the HCWs were stratified by professional group and, in five studies, by working area or exposure. Ten studies examined only a single professional group.

In 33 out of 57 studies, population-based controls, consisting mainly of blood donors, were used. A hospital control group was used in 18 studies. Ciorlia and Zanetta[38] used a population-

Review

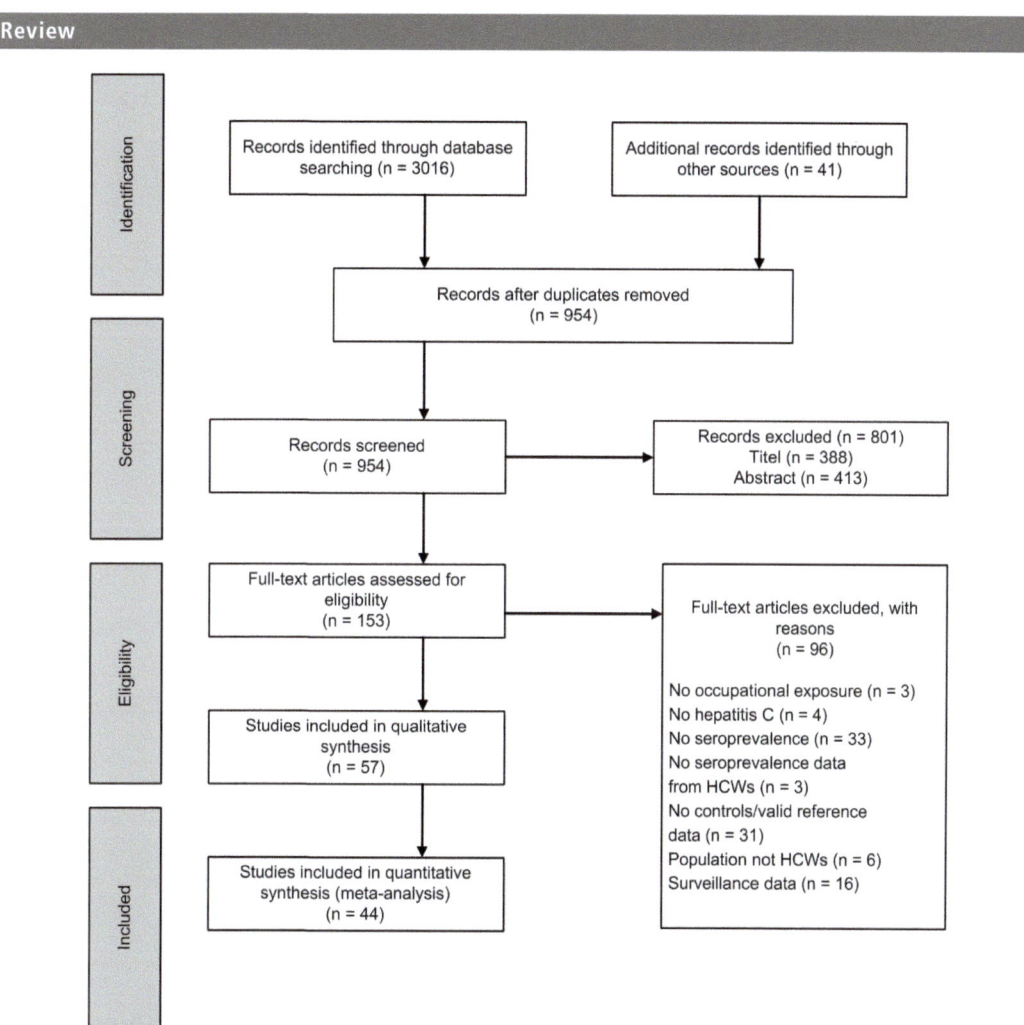

Figure 1 Selection process. HCWs, health care workers.

based and a hospital control group. Four studies used a population control and several other control groups, including risk groups such as dialysis patients and men who have sex with men.

Study design and quality
Fifty-one studies had a retrospective design and six a prospective design.[24–29] The annual incidence was reported in two studies only. According to Puro et al,[24] the rate was 0.1%; and 0.15% according to Cooper et al.[26]

The methodological quality was rated as high in seven studies, as moderate in 33 studies and as poor in 17 studies.

HCV detection
A HCV confirmation test was performed in 37 studies. Five studies used the same test for the confirmation as for the first test. There were differences between the studies with respect to the quality of the tests used (table 2).

HCV exposure among HCWs—a qualitative summary of studies not included in the meta-analysis
Thirteen studies could not be included in the meta-analysis because of missing case numbers (table 2). Increased HCV seroprevalence in HCWs in comparison to population controls was found in four out of seven studies of moderate methodological quality and in three out of six studies of low methodological quality. Cooper et al,[26] Goetz et al[53] and Zaaijer et al[66] studied employees stratified by their exposure risk. All seropositive employees worked in areas with high exposure to blood contact (eg, dialysis, blood bank, laboratory), or reported prior NSI.[26] With the exception of Mijakoski et al,[73] all controls were from reference sources.

Meta-analysis
The main results are shown as plots in figure 2. Further results of pooling analyses and subgroup analyses are summarised in online supplementary table S3.

Table 2 Characteristics of studies included

Author/year	Country	Period	HCV tests	HCWs	n (n+)	Prevalence %	Controls	n (n+)	Prevalence %	Study quality (scores)*
Prospective studies										
Puro 1995[24]	Italy	1992–1993	Anti-HCV 2, enzyme immunoassay RIBA 2	S	3073 (67)	2.2	Pr	11 000 (19)	1.7	High (8)[1–4 6–8]
Maillard 1996[25]	France	1992–1993	ELISA 2, PCR	S	236 (7)	2.9	H	305 (2)	0.7	Moderate (6)[1 2 5 7 8]
Cooper†1992[26]	USA	NA	EIA RIBA 2	S‡	243 (4)	1.6	Pr	–	0.4–1.4	Moderate (6)[2 4 7 8]
Ahmetagic 2006[27]	Bosnia and Herzegovina	2003–2005	ELISA 3, HCV-RNA	S	1699 (6)	0.4	P	2000 (4)	0.2	Low (4)[1 2 5 8]
Daw 2002[28]	Libya	1999–2001	ELISA	M, NS, CS‡	459 (9)	2	PS§	1200 (14)	1.2	Low (4)[1 2 5 8]
Mihaly† 2001[29]	Hungary	1986–1998	EIA 2, EIA 3, RIBA 3, PCR		477 (13)	2.7	Pr	–	0.73–1	Low (4)[1 2 8]
Retrospective studies										
Gershon 2007[30]	USA	1999–2000	HCV 2, RIBA 3	S	216 (4)	1.9	H	94 (3)	3.2	High (9)[1–8]
Ozsoy 2003[31]	Turkey	1998–2000	Anti-HCV 3 IL, INNOTEST 3, RT-PCR, ELISA	S	702 (2)	0.3	P	5670 (23)	0.4	High (9)[1–8]
Klein 1991[32]	USA	1985–1987	ELISA 1, RIBA	D	456 (8)	1.8	H	723 (1)	0.1	High (9)[1–8]
Sermoneta-Gertel 2001[33]	Israel	1995–1997	ELISA 3, RIBA 3	NS	3657 (34)	0.9	H	630 (3)	0.5	High (8)[1–6 8]
Thomas 1996[34]	USA	1991	ELISA 1 or ELISA 2, RIBA	NS	943 (7)	0.7	P	104,239 (417)	0.4	High (8)[1–5 7 8]
Struve 1994[35]	Sweden	NA	EIA 2, Supplementary test	M, NS, L¶	797 (5)	0.6	H	83 (1)	1.2	High (8)[1–5 7 8]
Braczkowska 2006[36]	Poland	2003–2004	ELISA 3,Western blot LIA HCV Ab3	MS	558 (8)	1.4	P	510 (2)	0.4	Moderate (7)[1–3 5 6 8]
Fisker 2004[37]	Denmark	1998	HCV 3, RIBA, PCR	S	960 (2)	0.2	P	479 (0)	–	Moderate (7)[1–5 8]
Ciorlia 2007[38]	Brazil	1994–1999	ELISA 2	S	1433 (25)	1.7	H, P	872 (4) 2583 (6)	1.3 0.2	Moderate (7)[1–6 8]
Moens 2000[39]	Belgium	1996–1997	EIA 3, Matrix Abbott und LIA, PCR	S‡	4480 (21)	0.4	H	426 (0)	–	Moderate (7)[1–3 6–8]
Thorburn 2001[40]	Scotland	1994–1996	ELISA 3, PCR, RIBA-3	S, D	10,654 (27)	0.3	H	471 (3)	0.6	Moderate (7)[1–3 5 7 8]
Djeriri 1996[41]	France	1993–1994	EIA 2 RIBA2	S	283 (2)	0.7	H	93 (0)	–	Moderate (7)[1–3 5 6 8]
Villate 1993[42]	Spain	1991–1992	ELISA 2, PCR, RIBA 2	M, L, NS¶	874 (14)	1.6	P	547 (2)	0.4	Moderate (7)[1–5 8]
Montella 2005[43]	Italy	1991	ELISA 1,ELISA new generation	M, NS, L¶	578 (32)	5.5	H	91 (6)	6.6	Moderate (7)[2 4–6 8]
Kaabia 2009[44]	Tunisia	2005	ELISA Murex 4, ELISA AxSYM Abbott	M, L, P, Mw¶	737 (9)	1.2	H	104 (0)	–	Moderate (6)[1–3 5 8]
Irani-Hakime 2001[45]	Lebanon	1999	SM-HCV rapid test, MEIA HCV 3, PCR	S	502 (2)	0.4	P	600 (1)	0.2	Moderate (6)[2 4 5 8]
Campello 2001[46]	Italy	1989–1990	ELISA, HCV neutralisation test	S	407 (5)	1.2	P	253 (2)	0.8	Moderate (6)[2 4 5 8]
Polish 1993[47]	USA	1983	Anti-HCV 1 Abbott, HCV neutralisation assay Abbott	S	1350 (22)	1.6	H	257 (1)	0.4	Moderate (6)[2 5 6 8]
Perez Trallero 1992[48]	Spain	NA	ELISA 2, RIBA 2	S	251 (4)	1.6	P	377 (8)	2.1	Moderate (6)[1 2 4 5 8]
Takahama 2005[49]	Brazil	NA	ELISA 3, PCR, AxSym Abbott 3	D	267 (1)	0.4	P	88,241 (304)	0.3	Moderate (6)[2 4 7 8]
Trevisan 1999[50]	Italy	NA	EIA, RIBA 3	S	809 (9)	1.1	H	408 (8)	2	Moderate (6)[2 4 5 8]
Webert 2001[51]	Switzerland	1999	EIA, EIA3, PCR, Immunoblot	D, DS	1056 (1)	0.1	Pr	–	0.5–1	Moderate (6)[2 4 7 8]
Shapiro† 1996[52]	USA	1991	Immunoassay 1, supplementary neutralisation assay	M	3262 (27)	0.8	Pr	–	0.09–0.36	Moderate(6)[2 4 7 8]
Goetz† 1995[53]	USA	NA	EIA 2, RIBA 2, Ortho, PCR	M, D, NS, L‡	241 (5)	1.3	Pr	–	0.3	Moderate (6)[2 4 7 8]
Ahmed 2012[54]	Pakistan	2007–2009	ETI-AB-HCV-4	S	41 (7)	17.1	P	1959 (103)	5.3	Moderate (5)[4–8]
Fischer 2000[55]	USA	1998	PCR	S	502 (0)	–	H	926 (2)	0.2	Moderate (5)[2 5 7 8]
De Mercato 1996[56]	Italy	1995	RIBA 2	S	472 (12)	2.5	P	285 (8)	2.8	Moderate (5)[2 4 5 8]

Continued

Westermann C, et al. Occup Environ Med 2015;72:880–888. doi:10.1136/oemed-2015-102879

Table 2 Continued

Author/year	Country	Period	HCV tests	HCWs	n (n+)	Prevalence %	Controls	n (n+)	Prevalence %	Study quality (scores)*
Olubuyide 1997[57]	Nigeria	1995	HCV 3-enzyme Immunoassay Murex	M, D	75 (8)	10.7	P	25 (3)	12	Moderate (5)[1 2 4 7 8]
Al-Sohaibani 1995[58]	Saudi Arabia	1992–1994	UBI HCV EIA, RIBA or LiaTEK HCV 3	M, MS¶	330 (8)	2.4	P	292 (5)	1.7	Moderate (5)[1 2 5 8]
Soni 1993[59]	South Africa	1991	EIA 2, EIA 2, Abbott neutralisation EIA	NS	212 (0)	–	P§	35 685 (92)	0.3	Moderate (5)[2 5 8]
Oguchi 1992[60]	Japan	1989	ELISA 1 or 2,	S	150 (3)	2	P	704 (7)	1	Moderate (5)[1 2 4 5 8]
Nakashima 1993[61]	Japan	1987–1988	ELISA, RIBA	S	1097 (11)	1	P	526 (5)	1	Moderate (5)[1 2 5 8]
Fujiyama 1992[62]	Japan	NA	ELISA anti-C100	S	152 (1)	0.7	P	919 (14)	1.5	Moderate (5)[1 2 5 8]
Germanaud** 1994[63]	France	NA	ELISA 2, RIBA 2	S	430 (4)	0.9	H	180 (3)	1.7	Moderate (5)[1 2 5 8]
Jindal† 2006[64]	India	2003	Hep-Chex C	S	100 (4)	4	Pr	–	1.6	Moderate (5)[1 2–4 8]
Kuo† 1993[65]	Taiwan	1990–1991	EIA 1, EIA 2, PCR	D	461 (3)	0.7	Pr	–	1	Moderate (5)[1 2 4 8]
Zaaijer† 2012[66]	The Netherlands	2000–2009	AxSYM HCV, RIBA 3, PCR	S‡	729 (1)	0.1	Pr	–	0.6	Moderate (5)[1 2 7 8]
Zuckerman† 1994[67]	Scotland	1986, 1991	EIA 2, RIBA 2	S	1053 (3)	0.3	Pr	–	0.3	Low (4)[1 2 8]
Jochen** 1992[68]	Germany	1992	EIA 2, Immunoblot 2	S	1033 (6)	0.6	P	2113 (5)	0.2	Low (4)[2 5 8]
El Gohary 1995[69]	Egypt	1990–1992	EIA 2	S	78 (6)	7.7	P§	271 (39)	14.4	Low (4)[1 2 5 8]
Polywka 1991[70]	Germany	NA	ELISA	S	217 (6)	2.8	P	500 (2)	0.4	Low (4)[1 2 5 8]
Hindy 1995[71]	Egypt	NA	ELISA, Abbott, ALT	DS	70 (1)	1.4	H	35 (6)	17.1	Low (4)[1 4 8]
Khan 2011[72]	Pakistan	NA	Immunochromatography test, PCR	NS	794 (34)	4.3	H	30 (0)	–	Low (4)[1 2 4 8]
Mijakoski† 2012[73]	Macedonia	NA	anti-HCV Ab	NS	54 (0)	–	H	32 (0)	–	Low (4)[1 4 5 8]
Kondili 2007[74]	Albania	NA	EIA 3	S	460 (3)	0.7	H	22 (0)	–	Low (3)[1 5 8]
Libanore** 1992[75]	Italy	NA	Immunoassay	S	1008 (41)	4.1	Pr	3572 (34)	1	Low (4)[1 2 5 8]
Mujeeb† 1998[76]	Pakistan	NA	EIA	S	114 (5)	4.4	Pr	–	0.7	Low (4)[1 2 4 8]
Sarkari† 2012[77]	Iran	2009–2010	ELISA 3	S	212 (9)	4.2	Pr	–	0.1–0.9	Low (4)[1 2 7 8]
Vardas 2002[78]	South Africa	1996	ELISA 3, PCR	S	362 (7)	1.9	H	37 (0)	0.2	Low (4)[1 2 8]
Shoaeit 2012[79]	Iran	2010	ELISA	L	203 (0)	–	Pr	–	0.2	Low (3)[1 2 8]
De Luca** 1992[80]	Italy	1990	NA	S	945 (45)	4.8	P§	3575 (39)	1.1	Low (2)[2 5]

() In bold letters: cases confirmed by second test.
*Fulfilled item for quality assessment—see table 1.
†Not included in meta-analysis.
‡Stratified by working area/exposure.
§Further control groups NA.
¶Stratified by professional groups.
**Editor letter.

CS, cleaning staff; D, medical dental staff; DS, dental staff (Medical and Non-Medical); EIA, enzyme immunoassay; H, hospital controls; HCV, viral hepatitis C; HCWs, healthcare workers; L, laboratory staff; M, medical staff; MS, medical students; Mw, midwives; NA, not available; NS, nursing staff; P, population-based controls; Pr, reference data on population-based controls; RIBA, the recombinant immunoblot assay; S, staff/ HCWs.

Westermann C, et al. Occup Environ Med 2015;72:880–888. doi:10.1136/oemed-2015-102879

A total of 44 studies were included in the pooled analysis (seven high quality studies, 26 moderate quality studies and 11 low quality studies—table 2). The pooled analysis of all studies showed a significantly increased OR of 1.5 (95% CI 1.15 to 2.06) for a HCV infection among HCWs compared to controls, with significant evidence of heterogeneity (χ^2=110.8, p<0.001,

I^2=61, see online supplementary table S3). The increased prevalence of HCV infection in HCWs was also observed in the 14 studies with high and moderate methodological quality, using population control groups and confirmatory tests (OR 1.6; 95% CI 1.03 to 2.42, no evidence of heterogeneity, figure 2).

After stratification by publication period, HCWs were found to have a statistically significant increased prevalence of HCV infection in the period 1989–2000 compared with all controls (OR 1.3; 95% CI 1.09 to 1.63). For the period 2000–2014, the pooled effect estimate was the same, but without a statistically significant increase (OR 1.3; 95% CI 0.89 to 2.02). As there are only a few current studies, it was not possible to conduct a test for time trend by subgroups (see online supplementary table S3).

The following analyses were based on high and moderate quality studies only.

Study region

Pooled analysis of studies from countries with comparably low HCV prevalence in Europe (Belgium, Denmark, France, Scotland, Sweden) and the USA showed a significantly increased prevalence of HCV infection in HCWs compared with controls (OR 2.1; 95% CI 1.31 to 3.42, figure 2). Further stratification by population-based controls could not be performed because of considerable variability between the studies (I^2=70). Pooled analysis of Japanese studies showed no increased HCV prevalence in HCWs (OR 1.1). Stratification of studies from the other countries by individual regions resulted in a statistically significant increased HCV prevalence in HCWs only for North Africa, the Middle East and South Asia (OR 1.9; 95% CI 1.10 to 3.15), compared to controls (see online supplementary table S3).

Gender

Six studies reported anti-HCV prevalence stratified by gender. By pooling studies using population-based controls with confirmatory tests, a significantly increased prevalence was observed only for male HCWs (women OR 1.5; 95% CI 0.45 to 5.24; men OR 3.1; 95% CI 1.21 to 7.99).

Professions

Medical staff: For medical personnel, pooled analysis of studies with confirmatory tests gave an OR of 2.7 (95% CI 1.65 to 4.51, figure 2). For medical staff excluding dentists, the OR was 2.2 (95% CI 1.30 to 3.77) for a HCV infection compared to population-based controls (see online supplementary material table S3).

Dental staff (medical and non-medical): Pooled analysis of studies with confirmatory tests gave an OR of 3.5 (95% CI 1.37 to 9.15, figure 2) for a HCV infection among dental staff compared to controls. Further stratification could not be performed because of considerable variability between the three studies.

Nursing staff: The pooled analysis of studies with confirmatory tests showed an OR of 1.7 (95% CI 0.86 to 3.31) for nursing staff compared to the population-based controls (see online supplementary table S3).

Laboratory staff: Pooled analysis of studies with confirmatory tests gave an increased OR of 2.2 (95% CI 1.10 to 4.39, figure 2) for a HCV infection in laboratory staff compared with all controls.

Professionals at high risk for blood contacts: Six sources contributed data on the following professions/working areas performing EPPs: surgeons, midwives, microbiologists, pathologists, blood bank and dialysis staff. All studies were published before 2000. The pooled analysis shows a statistically significant increased OR of 2.3 (95% CI 1.51 to 3.54) for a HCV infection

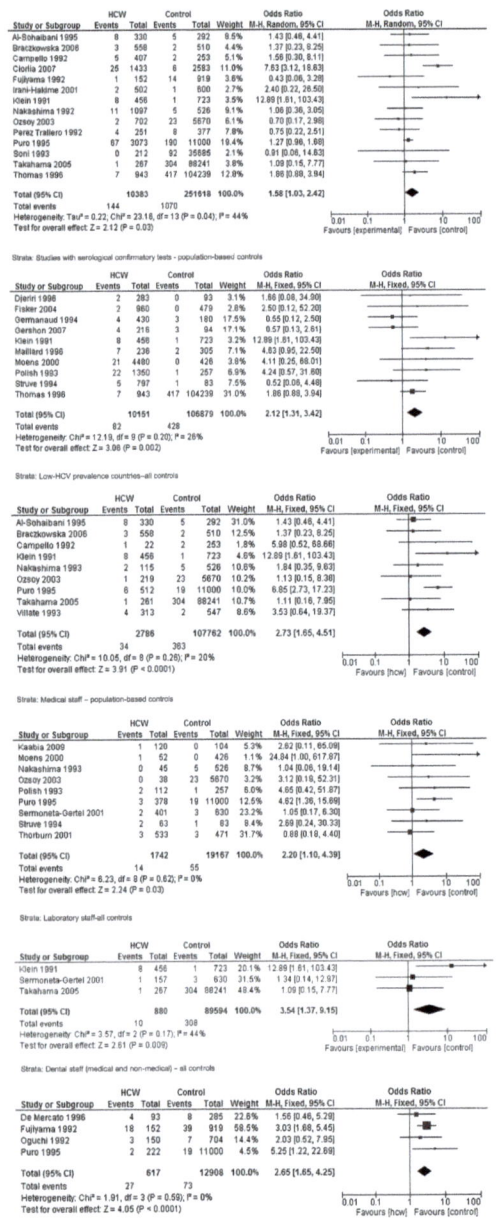

Figure 2 Forest plots of high and moderate quality studies on hepatitis C among healthcare workers. HCWs, health care workers.

among HCWs compared with all controls and of 2.7 (95% CI 1.84 to 5.53, figure 2) compared to population-based controls.

Heterogeneity and sensitivity analysis

Heterogeneity was present when pooling all studies. Pooling the studies with high and moderate methodological quality only, reduced heterogeneity. Further stratification was performed related to performance of confirmatory tests. In addition, individual studies were then sequentially excluded from the analysis in order to verify their influence on the pooled estimate.

Publication bias

The funnel plot did not show evidence of publication bias (see online supplementary figure S3), nor did Egger's linear regression show significant evidence of funnel plot asymmetry (intercept 0.19, 90% CI 0.33 to 0.71, p=0.47).

DISCUSSION

This is the first systematic review to perform a meta-analysis on the prevalence of HCV infection among HCWs in comparison to controls. The pooled analysis of high and moderate quality studies gave a statistically significant increase in OR of 1.6 for HCV infection among HCWs compared to population-based controls. Stratified pooled analysis of studies with confirmatory tests from countries with comparable low HCV prevalence also resulted in a statistically significant increase in OR for HCWs in comparison to controls (OR 2.1). Stratification by occupational groups demonstrated an increased prevalence among *medical staff* (OR 2.2), *laboratory staff* (OR 2.2) and *dental staff* (medical and non-medical, OR 3.5), compared to controls. However, due to the few studies found for dental staff, further stratification by profession could not be performed. In addition, the pooled effect estimated is mainly caused by one high quality study with a wide CI.[32] When the pooled analysis was stratified by *nursing staff*, no significant increase in OR was found. A differentiated examination of activity profile-related occupational hazards was carried out for this profession in only a few studies. This lack of differentiation may lead to underestimation of the occupational risk of infection due to exposure misclassification. This happens particularly when HCWs who are frequently exposed to blood while performing EPPs are examined in combination with less exposed HCWs in the same job category. Pooled analysis for each individual group—such as cleaning staff—was not possible as the studies were few and their methods heterogeneous in design, HCWs examined, serological testing and controls. This diversity is the main reason for the lack of consensus in the assessment of the occupational risk of HCV infection in HCWs.[81–83] Additionally, it is difficult to quantify the occupational risk given to a specific profession, such as for laboratory staff, as there is no systematic record of how exposure depends on the activity.[84] To estimate HCV prevalence in HCWs due to specific work profiles, we conducted an exemplary pooled analysis of professions that performed EPPs in accordance with the criteria of Trevisan et al.[50] The pooled analysis shows a significantly increased OR of 2.7 for these employees in comparison to the population-based controls. However, the results of this subgroup analysis are based only on studies published before 2000. The assessment of personal risk factors for a HCV infection was not performed consistently in the investigated studies, particularly in studies published earlier. Those examinations were conducted prior to the Needlestick Safety and Prevention Act (NSPA). Both in the USA and in Europe, guidelines have been issued since 2000 that aim to prevent exposure to blood, for example, from NSI.[6 85]

The results of studies that could not be included in the quantitative analysis did not conflict with the results of the meta-analysis. Professions that performed EPPs are exposed to NSI, with a HCV transmission rate of 1.8% after an NSI according to Henderson,[83] Riddell and Sherrard,[86] and Baldo et al.[87] The results of an American multicentre study performed in 2006 showed that occupational exposure was greater in male HCWs.[88] The authors observed that men were three times more frequently infected than their female colleagues. In this context, bivariate analysis showed that glove use when performing invasive work was significantly associated with the female gender. According to the reviews of Kubitschke et al[8] and Goniewicz et al,[89] NSIs were more frequent in inexperienced personnel. Current findings on the incidence of NSI in the health service show that nursing[6 88 90] and medical personnel[88] are the most frequently affected professional group. According to Butsashvili et al[88] the highest number of exposures to NSI is in dialysis work. The most recent research on dialysis staff (2006–2010) concluded that there had been no decrease in the number of observed NSIs suffered by staff.[6]

Strengths and limitations

This is the first meta-analysis to examine the prevalence of HCV infection in HCWs compared to controls. However, the mostly retrospective studies included some recent studies. In addition, older studies tend to report higher anti-HCV prevalence rates than more recent studies (as confirmed by Larney et al[91]). As there are only a few current studies, it was not possible to draw reliable conclusions about a time trend. Most of the population-based controls were blood donors. Individuals at risk of HCV infection in the general population were probably not included. The results of the studies that referred to reference populations must also be viewed critically. HCWs and controls may not have been tested under identical conditions. Few studies have examined how occupational hazards depend on the activity profile. This lack of differentiation may lead to underestimation of the occupational risk of infection for specific HCWs. So, the present results reveal a strong demand for further differentiated research.

Quality of serological testing

The quality of the confirmatory tests used clearly differs between individual studies. This is due to the development of better detection methods over time, the quality of the procedure or the fact that there is no fundamental difference between the antigens used in the screening and the confirmatory tests. Owing to the limitations in the sensitivity of the first anti-HCV tests (false negatives), earlier studies tended to underestimate seroprevalence. In contrast, limitations in specificity lead to false positive results. This may result in non-differential misclassification, which again is most likely to lead to decreased effect estimates.

Assessment of personal risk factors

The personal risk factors for HCV infection were not recorded consistently in the studies. The risk factors, such as use of injected drugs and injury-prone sex (men with men) were not collected in many studies, especially the earlier ones. The 1998 report of the US Center for Disease Control and Prevention (CDC) on the known risks of HCV infection identified drug use and injury-prone sex as the most common causes.[15] Of the six studies that allow stratification by gender, only two examined these confounding factors, which are associated with a higher risk of non-occupationally acquired HCV infection, especially among men.[32 36]

CONCLUSION

This meta-analysis shows a statistically significant increase in the prevalence of HCV infection in HCWs compared to controls. Medical and laboratory personnel, and staff members who perform EPPs, are particularly affected. For other professions, no adequate calculation of a pooled estimate was possible. Prevalence of HCV infection has probably decreased since 2000, due to improved prevention. However, this needs to be investigated further. To analyse HCWs' occupational risk of infection, prospective studies are needed that focus on HCWs in terms of specific work profiles bearing in mind the importance of assessment of personal risk factors for infection. Contact with blood, for example, from NSI, is associated with a risk of infection and continues to be the major threat to the health of HCWs. Targeted prevention measures must be based on the epidemiological detection and evaluation of work-related accidents. Readily accessible reporting and treatment procedures, and the use of safe practices for working with blood, can help to minimise occupational exposure.

Collaborators Melanie Harling.

Contributors CW conceived the study protocol, performed the study selection, data extraction, quality assessment and statistical analysis, and wrote the first draft of the manuscript. CP was involved in performing data extraction, quality assessment and statistical analysis and made substantial contributions toward revising the first draft. BL performed the study selection and assessment, and made substantial contributions towards revising the first draft. ML made substantial contributions toward revising the first draft. AN coordinated the study, amended the study protocol, assisted in study selection and statistical analysis, and made substantial contributions toward revising the first draft.

Competing interests None declared.

Provenance and peer review Not commissioned; externally peer reviewed.

Open Access This is an Open Access article distributed in accordance with the Creative Commons Attribution Non Commercial (CC BY-NC 4.0) license, which permits others to distribute, remix, adapt, build upon this work non-commercially, and license their derivative works on different terms, provided the original work is properly cited and the use is non-commercial. See: http://creativecommons.org/licenses/by-nc/4.0/

REFERENCES

1 World Health Organization. *Prevention and control of viral hepatitis infection: framework for global action.* Geneva, 2012:28.
2 Askarian M, Yadollahi M, Kuochak F, *et al.* Precautions for health care workers to avoid hepatitis B and C virus infection. *Int J Occup Environ Med* 2011;2:191–8.
3 Te HS, Jensen DM. Epidemiology of hepatitis B and C viruses: a global overview. *Clin Liver Dis* 2010;14:1–21, vii.
4 Deuffic-Burban S, Delarocque-Astagneau E, Abiteboul D, *et al.* Blood-borne viruses in health care workers: prevention and management. *J Clin Virol* 2011;52:4–10.
5 Nienhaus A, Kesavachandran C, Wendeler D, *et al.* Infectious diseases in healthcare workers—an analysis of the standardised data set of a German compensation board. *J Occup Med Toxicol* 2012;7:8.
6 Elseviers MM, Arias-Guillen M, Gorke A, *et al.* Sharps injuries amongst healthcare workers: review of incidence, transmissions and costs. *J Ren Care* 2014;40:150–6.
7 Himmelreich H, Rabenau HF, Rindermann M, *et al.* The management of needlestick injuries. *Dtsch Arztebl Int* 2013;110:61–7.
8 Kubitschke A, Bahr MJ, Aslan N, *et al.* Induction of hepatitis C virus (HCV)-specific T cells by needle stick injury in the absence of HCV-viraemia. *Eur J Clin Invest* 2007;37:54–64.
9 Sulkowski MS, Ray SC, Thomas DL. Needlestick transmission of hepatitis C. *JAMA* 2002;287:2406–13.
10 Yazdanpanah Y, De CG, Migueres B, *et al.* Risk factors for hepatitis C virus transmission to health care workers after occupational exposure: a European case-control study. *Clin Infect Dis* 2005;41:1423–30.
11 Wicker S, Rabenau HF, Haberl AE, *et al.* Blutübertragbare Infektionen und die schwangere Mitarbeiterin im Gesundheitswesen. Risiko und Präventionsmaßnahmen Blood-borne infections and the pregnant health care worker. Risks and preventive measures. *Chirurg* 2012;83:136–42.
12 Hofmann F, Kralj N, Beie M. Kanülenstichverletzungen im Gesundheitsdienst—Häufigkeiten, Ursachen und Präventionsstrategien Needle stick injuries in health care—frequency, causes und preventive strategies. *Gesundheitswesen* 2002;64:259–66.
13 Dulon M, Nienhaus A. Aktuelle Trends bei Infektionskrankheiten der Beschäftigten im Gesundheitsdienst—2008 bis 2012. In: Nienhaus A, ed. *RiRe—Risiken und Ressourcen in Gesundheitsdienst und Wohlfahrtspflege.* Heidelberg: Ecomed Medizin, 2014:27–40.
14 Stroup DF, Berlin JA, Morton SC, *et al.* Meta-analysis of observational studies in epidemiology: a proposal for reporting. Meta-analysis Of Observational Studies in Epidemiology (MOOSE) group. *JAMA* 2000;283:2008–12.
15 [No authors listed]. Public Health Service guidelines for the management of health-care worker exposures to HIV and recommendations for postexposure prophylaxis. Centers for Disease Control and Prevention. *MMWR Recomm Rep* 1998;47:1–33.
16 Downs SH, Black N. The feasibility of creating a checklist for the assessment of the methodological quality both of randomised and non-randomised studies of health care interventions. *J Epidemiol Community Health* 1998;52:377–84.
17 Loney PL, Chambers LW, Bennett KJ, *et al.* Critical appraisal of the health research literature: prevalence or incidence of a health problem. *Chronic Dis Can* 1998;19:170–6.
18 Higgins JPT, Green S, eds. *Cochran handbook for systematic reviews of interventions 4.2.6.* Chichester, UK: John Wiley & Sons, 2006.
19 Slim K, Nini E, Forestier D, *et al.* Methodological index for non-randomized studies (minors): development and validation of a new instrument. *ANZ J Surg* 2003;73:712–16.
20 Vandenbroucke JP, von Elm E, Altman DG, *et al.* Strengthening the Reporting of Observational Studies in Epidemiology (STROBE): explanation and elaboration. *PLoS Med* 2007;4:e297.
21 Hahne SJ, Veldhuijzen IK, Wiessing L, *et al.* Infection with hepatitis B and C virus in Europe: a systematic review of prevalence and cost-effectiveness of screening. *BMC Infect Dis* 2013;13:181.
22 Mohd Hanafiah K, Groeger J, Flaxman AD, *et al.* Global epidemiology of hepatitis C virus infection: new estimates of age-specific antibody to HCV seroprevalence. *Hepatology* 2013;57:1333–42.
23 Egger M, Davey Smith G, Schneider M, *et al.* Bias in meta-analysis detected by a simple, graphical test. *BMJ* 1997;315:629–34.
24 Puro V, Petrosillo N, Ippolito G, *et al.* Occupational hepatitis C virus infection in Italian health care workers. Italian Study Group on Occupational Risk of Bloodborne Infections. *Am J Public Health* 1995;85:1272–5.
25 Maillard MF, Poynard T, Dubreuil P, *et al.* Prevalence of serum anti-hepatitis C virus antibodies and risk factors of contamination in the personnel of a hospital in the Paris region. A prospective survey. *Gastroenterol Clin Biol* 1996;20:1053–7.
26 Cooper BW, Krusell A, Tilton RC, *et al.* Seroprevalence of antibodies to hepatitis C virus in high-risk hospital personnel. *Infect Control Hosp Epidemiol* 1992;13:82–5.
27 Ahmetagic S, Muminhodzic K, Cickusic E, *et al.* Hepatitis C infection in risk groups. *Bosn J Basic Med Sci* 2006;6:13–17.
28 Daw MA, Elkaber MA, Drah AM, *et al.* Prevalence of hepatitis C virus antibodies among different populations of relative and attributable risk. *Saudi Med J* 2002;23:1356–60.
29 Mihaly I, Telegdy L, Ibranyi E, *et al.* Prevalence, genotype distribution and outcome of hepatitis C infections among the employees of the Hungarian Central Hospital for infectious diseases. *J Hosp Infect* 2001;49:239–44.
30 Gershon RR, Sherman M, Mitchell C, *et al.* Prevalence and risk factors for bloodborne exposure and infection in correctional healthcare workers. *Infect Control Hosp Epidemiol* 2007;28:24–30.
31 Ozsoy MF, Oncul O, Cavuslu S, *et al.* Seroprevalences of hepatitis B and C among health care workers in Turkey. *J Viral Hepat* 2003;10:150–6.
32 Klein RS, Freeman K, Taylor PE, *et al.* Occupational risk for hepatitis C virus infection among New York City dentists. *Lancet* 1991;338:1539–42.
33 Sermoneta-Gertel S, Donchin M, Adler R, *et al.* Hepatitis c virus infection in employees of a large university hospital in Israel. *Infect Control Hosp Epidemiol* 2001;22:754–61.
34 Thomas DL, Gruninger SE, Siew C, *et al.* Occupational risk of hepatitis C infections among general dentists and oral surgeons in North America. *Am J Med* 1996;100:41–5.
35 Struve J, Aronsson B, Frenning B, *et al.* Prevalence of antibodies against hepatitis C virus infection among health care workers in Stockholm. *Scand J Gastroenterol* 1994;29:360–2.
36 Braczkowska B, Kowalskan M, Zejda JE, *et al.* Prevalence and basic determinants of hepatitis C antibodies in medical students in Katowice, Poland. *Przegl Lek* 2006;63:539–42.
37 Fisker N, Mygind LH, Krarup HB, *et al.* Blood borne viral infections among Danish health care workers--frequent blood exposure but low prevalence of infection. *Eur J Epidemiol* 2004;19:61–7.
38 Ciorlia LA, Zanetta DM. Hepatitis C in health care professionals: prevalence and association with risk factors. *Rev Saude Publica* 2007;41:229–35.
39 Moens G, Vranckx R, de Greef L, *et al.* Prevalence of hepatitis C antibodies in a large sample of Belgian healthcare workers. *Infect Control Hosp Epidemiol* 2000;21:209–12.

Review

40 Thorburn D, Dundas D, McCruden EA, *et al*. A study of hepatitis C prevalence in healthcare workers in the West of Scotland. *Gut* 2001;48:116–20.
41 Djeriri K, Fontana L, Laurichesse H, *et al*. Seroprevalence of markers of viral hepatitis A, B and C in hospital personnel at the Clermont-Ferrand University Hospital Center. *Presse Med* 1996;25:145–50.
42 Villate JI, Corral J, Aguirre C, *et al*. Hepatitis C virus antibodies in hospital personnel. *Med Clin (Barc)* 1993;100:766–9.
43 Montella M, Crispo A, Grimaldi M, *et al*. An assessment of hepatitis C virus infection among health-care workers of the National Cancer Institute of Naples, Southern Italy. *Eur J Public Health* 2005;15:467–9.
44 Kaabia N, Ben JE, Hannachi N, *et al*. Prevalence of hepatitis C virus among health care workers in central Tunisia. *Med Mal Infect* 2009;39:66–7.
45 Irani-Hakime N, Aoun J, Khoury S, *et al*. Seroprevalence of hepatitis C infection among health care personnel in Beirut, Lebanon. *Am J Infect Control* 2001;29:20–3.
46 Campello C, Majori S, Poli A, *et al*. Prevalence of HCV antibodies in health-care workers from northern Italy. *Infection* 1992;20:224–6.
47 Polish LB, Tong MJ, Co RL, *et al*. Risk factors for hepatitis C virus infection among health care personnel in a community hospital. *Am J Infect Control* 1993;21:196–200.
48 Perez Trallero E, Cilla G, Alcorta M, *et al*. Low risk of acquiring the hepatitis C virus for the health personnel. *Med Clin (Barc)* 1992;99:609–11.
49 Takahama AJ, Tatsch F, Tannus G, *et al*. Hepatitis C: incidence and knowledge among Brazilian dentists. *Community Dent Health* 2005;22:184–7.
50 Trevisan A, Bicciato F, Fanelli G, *et al*. Risk of hepatitis C virus infection in a population exposed to biological materials. *Am J Ind Med* 1999;35:532–5.
51 Weber C, Coller-Schaub D, Fried R, *et al*. Low prevalence of hepatitis C virus antibody among Swiss dental health care workers. *J Hepatol* 2001;34:963–4.
52 Shapiro CN, Tokars JI, Chamberland ME. Use of the hepatitis-B vaccine and infection with hepatitis B and C among orthopaedic surgeons. The American Academy of Orthopaedic Surgeons Serosurvey Study Committee. *J Bone Joint Surg Am* 1996;78:1791–800.
53 Goetz AM, Ndimbie OK, Wagener MM, *et al*. Prevalence of hepatitis C infection in health care workers affiliated with a liver transplant center. *Transplantation* 1995;59:990–4.
54 Ahmed F, Irving WL, Anwar M, *et al*. Prevalence and risk factors for hepatitis C virus infection in Kech District, Balochistan, Pakistan: most infections remain unexplained. A cross-sectional study. *Epidemiol Infect* 2012;140:716–23.
55 Fischer LR, Tope DH, Conboy KS, *et al*. Screening for hepatitis C virus in a health maintenance organization. *Arch Intern Med* 2000;160:1665–73.
56 De Mercato R, Guarnaccia D, Ciannella G, *et al*. Hepatitis C virus among health care workers. *Minerva Med* 1996;87:501–4.
57 Olubuyide IO, Ola SO, Aliyu B, *et al*. Prevalence and epidemiological characteristics of hepatitis B and C infections among doctors and dentists in Nigeria. *East Afr Med J* 1997;74:357–61.
58 al-Sohaibani MO, al-Sheikh EH, al-Ballal SJ, *et al*. Occupational risk of hepatitis B and C infections in Saudi medical staff. *J Hosp Infect* 1995;31:143–7.
59 Soni PN, Tait DR, Kenoyer DG, *et al*. Hepatitis C virus antibodies among risk groups in a South African area endemic for hepatitis B virus. *J Med Virol* 1993;40:65–8.
60 Oguchi H, Miyasaka M, Tokunaga S, *et al*. Hepatitis virus infection (HBV and HCV) in eleven Japanese hemodialysis units. *Clin Nephrol* 1992;38:36–43.
61 Nakashima K, Kashiwagi S, Hayashi J, *et al*. Low prevalence of hepatitis C virus infection among hospital staff and acupuncturists in Kyushu, Japan. *J Infect* 1993;26:17–25.
62 Fujiyama S, Kawano S, Sato S, *et al*. Prevalence of hepatitis C virus antibodies in hemodialysis patients and dialysis staff. *Hepatogastroenterology* 1992;39:161–5.
63 Germanaud J, Barthez JP, Causse X. The occupational risk of hepatitis C infection among hospital employees. *Am J Public Health* 1994;84:122.
64 Jindal N, Jindal M, Jilani N, *et al*. Seroprevalence of hepatitis C virus (HCV) in health care workers of a tertiary care centre in New Delhi. *Indian J Med Res* 2006;123:179–80.
65 Kuo MY, Hahn LJ, Hong CY, *et al*. Low prevalence of hepatitis C virus infection among dentists in Taiwan. *J Med Virol* 1993;40:10–13.
66 Zaaijer HL, Appelman P, Frijstein G. Hepatitis C virus infection among transmission-prone medical personnel. *Eur J Clin Microbiol Infect Dis* 2012;31:1473–7.
67 Zuckerman J, Clewley G, Griffiths P, *et al*. Prevalence of hepatitis C antibodies in clinical health-care workers. *Lancet* 1994;343:1618–20.
68 Jochen AB. Occupationally acquired hepatitis C virus infection. *Lancet* 1992;339:304.
69 el Gohary A, Hassan A, Nooman Z, *et al*. High prevalence of hepatitis C virus among urban and rural population groups in Egypt. *Acta Trop* 1995;59:155–61.
70 Polywka S, Laufs R. Hepatitis C virus antibodies among different groups at risk and patients with suspected non-A, non-B hepatitis. *Infection* 1991;19:81–4.
71 Hindy AM, Abdelhaleem ES, Aly RH. Hepatitis B and C viruses among Egyptian dentists. *Egypt Dent J* 1995;41:1217–26.
72 Khan S, Attaullah S, Ayaz S, *et al*. Molecular epidemiology of HCV among health care workers of khyber pakhtunkhwa. *Virol J* 2011;8:105.
73 Mijakoski D, Karadzinska-Bislimovska J, Stikova E, *et al*. Occupational sharp injuries and biological markers of hepatitis B and hepatitis C viral infection in nurses. *Macedonian J Med Sci* 2012;4:417–27.
74 Kondili LA, Ulqinaku D, Hajdini M, *et al*. Hepatitis B virus infection in health care workers in Albania: a country still highly endemic for HBV infection. *Infection* 2007;35:94–7.
75 Libanore M, Bicocchi R, Ghinelli F, *et al*. Prevalence of antibodies to hepatitis C virus in Italian health care workers. *Infection* 1992;20:50.
76 Mujeeb SA, Khatri Y, Khanani R. Frequency of parenteral exposure and seroprevalence of HBV, HCV, and HIV among operation room personnel. *J Hosp Infect* 1998;38:133–7.
77 Sarkari B, Eilami O, Khosravani A, *et al*. High prevalence of hepatitis C infection among high risk groups in Kohgiloyeh and Boyerahmad Province, Southwest Iran. *Arch Iran Med* 2012;15:271–4.
78 Vardas E, Ross MH, Sharp G, *et al*. Viral hepatitis in South African healthcare workers at increased risk of occupational exposure to blood-borne viruses. *J Hosp Infect* 2002;50:6–12.
79 Shoaei P, Lotfi N, Hassannejad R, *et al*. Seroprevalence of hepatitis C infection among laboratory health care workers in Isfahan, Iran. *Int J Prev Med* 2012;3:S146–9.
80 De Luca M, Ascione A, Vacca C, *et al*. Are health-care workers really at risk of HCV infection? *Lancet* 1992;339:1364–5.
81 Sepkowitz KA. Occupationally acquired infections in health care workers. Part II. *Ann Intern Med* 1996;125:917–28.
82 Lanphear BP. Transmission and control of bloodborne viral hepatitis in health care workers. *Occup Med (Lond)* 1997;12:717–30.
83 Henderson DK. Managing occupational risks for hepatitis C transmission in the health care setting. *Clin Microbiol Rev* 2003;16:546–68.
84 Singh K. Laboratory-acquired infections. *Clin Infect Dis* 2009;49:142–7.
85 Phillips EK, Conaway MR, Jagger JC. Percutaneous injuries before and after the Needlestick Safety and Prevention Act. *N Engl J Med* 2012;366:670–1.
86 Riddell LA, Sherrard J. Blood-borne virus infection: the occupational risks. *Int J STD AIDS* 2000;11:632–9.
87 Baldo V, Baldovin T, Trivello R, *et al*. Epidemiology of HCV infection. *Curr Pharm Des* 2008;14:1646–54.
88 Butsashvili M, Kamkamidze G, Kajaia M, *et al*. Occupational exposure to body fluids among health care workers in Georgia. *Occup Med (Lond)* 2012;62:620–6.
89 Goniewicz M, Wloszczak-Szubzda A, Niemcewicz M, *et al*. Injuries caused by sharp instruments among healthcare workers--international and Polish perspectives. *Ann Agric Environ Med* 2012;19:523–7.
90 Shah SM, Bonauto D, Silverstein B, *et al*. Workers' compensation claims for needlestick injuries among healthcare workers in Washington State, 1996–2000. *Infect Control Hosp Epidemiol* 2005;26:775–81.
91 Larney S, Kopinski H, Beckwith CG, *et al*. Incidence and prevalence of hepatitis C in prisons and other closed settings: results of a systematic review and meta-analysis. *Hepatology* 2013;58:1215–24.

Westermann et al. Journal of Occupational Medicine and Toxicology (2016) 11:52
DOI 10.1186/s12995-016-0142-5

Journal of Occupational
Medicine and Toxicology

RESEARCH

Open Access

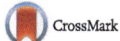

Hepatitis C among healthcare personnel: secondary data analyses of costs and trends for hepatitis C infections with occupational causes

Claudia Westermann[1]*, Madeleine Dulon[2], Dana Wendeler[2] and Albert Nienhaus[1,2]

Abstract

Background: Hepatitis C infection is a global public health issue. Chronic hepatitis C infection is associated with significant morbidity and mortality. The aim of this study is to describe the costs for occupationally-cased hepatitis C infections based on data from an accident insurance carrier.

Methods: This study is a secondary analysis based on the Database of a German Institution for Statutory Accident Insurance. The analysis is based on a sample of insured parties whose hepatitis C infections were recorded as occupational diseases between 1996 and 2013. The analysis is based on recognised hepatitis C cases and incorporates records registered between 1 January 2000 and 31 December 2014.

Results: Within the study period, the number of reported and recognised hepatitis C cases declined by 73 and 86% respectively. The majority of recognised hepatitis C cases ($n = 1.121$) were female, older than 40 years and were active in a medical nursing profession. In the study period, the costs came to a total of € 87.9 million, of which 60% was attributable to pension payments (€ 51,570,830) and around 15% was attributable to pharmaceutical and medicinal products (€ 12,978,318). Expenses for drugs exhibited heavy increases in 2012 (from around € 500,000– 800,000 to € 1.7 million) and 2014 (to € 2.5 million) in particular. Pension payments came to € 1.6 million in 2000 and rose continuously to over € 4 million in 2014. Expenses for occupational rehabilitation accounted for less than 1%.

Conclusions: For hepatitis C infections as an occupational disease, a considerable increase in costs has been observed in recent years, while the number of reports has declined heavily. This rise in costs is explained by the increase in pension payments and, since 2012, by a rise in the costs for drugs. The high costs of anti-viral therapies is offset by the potential for considerable treatment benefits. Healing the infection is expected to generate long-term cost savings for statutory accident insurance carriers, and also for social security systems.

Keywords: Hepatitis C virus, Occupational disease, Healthcare personnel, Burden of disease, Secondary data analysis

* Correspondence: c.westermann@uke.de
[1]University Medical Center Hamburg-Eppendorf (UKE), Center of Excellence
for Health Services Research in Nursing (CVcare), Hamburg, Germany
Full list of author information is available at the end of the article

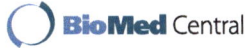

Publikation 2

Westermann *et al. Journal of Occupational Medicine and Toxicology* (2016) 11:52

Page 2 of 8

Background

The viral disease hepatitis C (HCV) is globally one of the most common infectious diseases. The hepatitis C RNA virus is transmitted from person to person, primarily through contact with infected blood while the skin or mucosa is also injured [1]. Healthcare personnel are at greater risk of HCV infection due to the nature of their occupational duties [2]. The progression of the infection is often non-specific, which is why the infection often remains undetected. Up to 85% of infections are chronic (HCV-RNA positive longer than six months). According to data from the World Health Organisation (WHO), around 150 million people globally have chronic hepatitis C (CHC); 700,000 people die each year as a result [1, 3, 4]. CHC is associated with a high level of morbidity and a diminished quality of life. Up to 68% of patients suffer from symptoms including fatigue, exhaustion, limited performance and subclinical cognitive impairment. CHC is also associated with an increased risk for developing cirrhosis of the liver and hepatocellular carcinoma [4, 5]. A variety of extrahepatic manifestations may also develop. The development of depression symptoms, diabetes mellitus and malignant lymphoproliferative disorders such as follicular non-Hodgkin lymphoma are associated with HCV. Several studies have also indicated impairment of certain central nervous functions and neurotransmission [4]. US scientists have calculated the costs for the US healthcare system associated with CHC on the basis of data from a private health insurance company. They (retrospectively) studied the insurance data of 53,796 CHC patients over a period of eight years (2002–2010), according to which the average cost attributable to CHC per patient, per year was $ 24,176 (approx. € 21,776). Stratified according to stages of the disease, these costs increase as the disease progresses, reaching their peak in patients with terminal cirrhosis of the liver ($ 59,995/€ 53,880 per patient, per year) [6]. According to estimates, the share of patients with manifest liver disease will quadruple over the next 20 years without effective treatment [7]. Due to the potentially severe progression of the disease and the high associated costs, successful treatment of CHC is important [3, 6, 7]. The use of second-generation direct anti-viral agents (DAAs) today provide promising treatment combinations. Treatment of a CHC infection is considered successful if RNA viruses (HCV-RNA) can no longer be detected in the blood between 12 and 24 weeks after treatment is concluded [4, 5, 8]. As initial publications have shown, interferon-free DAA treatments have achieved substantial sustained virological response rates (SVRs) of over 90% in both treatment-naive and treatment-experienced patients with CHC infections. Such treatments are shorter than previous interferon-based therapies, have fewer side effects, and are currently a recommended course of treatment for HCV infections [3, 4].

The purpose of this study is to illustrate the costs for occupational hepatitis C infections based on data of the Institution for Statutory Accident Insurance and Prevention in the Health and Welfare Services (Berufsgenossenschaft für Gesundheitsdienst und Wohlfahrtspflege, BGW) for the period from 2000 to 2014.

Methods

This study is reported in line with A Consensus German Reporting Standard for Secondary Data Analyses, Version 2 (STROSA) [9].

Secondary data from BGW were used to analyse the costs of occupational HCV infections. BGW's occupational disease routine data records (BK-DOK) were used as a data source.

Occupational disease procedure

In Germany, if there is reasonable cause to suspect an occupational disease (OD), physicians are required to submit a report. Reports of suspected ODs may also be submitted by health insurers, employers, representatives of company interests or parties insured with the statutory accident insurance carriers. The statutory accident insurance carriers will follow an investigative procedure to determine whether a disease is an OD as defined by the Occupational Disease Ordinance (*Berufskrankheiten-Verordnung*, BKV) (Section 9, para. 1 & 2 of the German Social Security Code VII). A fully documented connection must be established here between the insured activity and the damaging exposure. The disease must also be fully documented. There must be a probable causal relationship between the exposure and the disease.

In the case of infectious diseases, the exposure is often difficult to identify, which is why it is sufficient to prove that duties have been performed that are associated with an elevated risk of infection. The performance of surgery and contact with blood would be an example of such a hazardous activity with an elevated risk for blood-borne viral diseases. An occupational infectious disease can either be classified as an insurance claim without entitlement to pension disbursement (if the reduced work ability –RWA– is less than 20%), or an entitlement to pension disbursement can be recognised. If there is already a 10% RWA from a previous insurance claim, a new 10% RWA can give rise to a pension disbursement entitlement. In cases where the OD suspicion has not been proven, a rejection is issued.

Documentation of OD reports

The key features of an OD suspicion report are registered in a standardised fashion in BK-DOK. OD suspicion reports are fundamentally registered as reportable if there are indications of an infection. This applies irrespective of which decision is taken under insurance law

Westermann *et al. Journal of Occupational Medicine and Toxicology* (2016) 11:52

in the investigative procedure later. Because the investigative procedure is time-consuming and a decision may not be taken in the year of the OD report, the cases ruled upon in a given reporting year can contain suspicion reports from previous years.

Analysis

The analysis of the BK-DOK is based on data from insured parties whose HCV infections were reported as suspected ODs between 1996 and 2013. The sample was acquired from the "Insurance Claims" database, which contains not only fundamental personal data but also other details (including sociodemographic features such as sex, year of birth, industry, profession, diagnostic information, year of registration, first and most recent decision, year of decision, OD-triggering circumstances, insurance claim reference number, etc.) The "Compensation Payments" database provided data on expenses incurred on behalf of the insured for drugs and benefits related to medical and occupational rehabilitation.

Analysis of reduced work ability [RWA]

The RWA classification may change over the course of the disease, depending on the severity of the disease at any given time. The level of impairment and the dates on which it starts and ends are documented for each change

in RWA. The analysis of the RWA is based on data from 1996 to 2014 and relates to the first established RWA and the current RWA (as of 31 December 2014). For the presentation of changes in the RWA, CHC patients were sorted according to the current RWA (as of the analysis date) and grouped according to the year of registration of the OD (in five-year groups). Distribution of current RWAs in the respective accident registration periods is presented using percentiles.

Because data on compensation payments have only been collected and processed since 2000, only registrations falling between 1 January 2000 and 31 December 2014 are reflected. The registration titles were grouped and reduced from 100 down to nine categories. In order to represent changes in compensation payments, we have allocated costs to medical rehabilitation (medicines, pharmaceuticals, inpatient and outpatient treatment), occupational rehabilitation (phased return, retraining, etc.) and pension payments (Fig. 2). The results are presented descriptively (absolute and relative frequencies), and the incurred costs are added together over a reporting period of 15 years.

Data on insured parties is provided from within BGW by the Rehabilitation Coordination department. It is derived from the standardised occupational diseases records and is analysed in anonymised form. Data were acquired

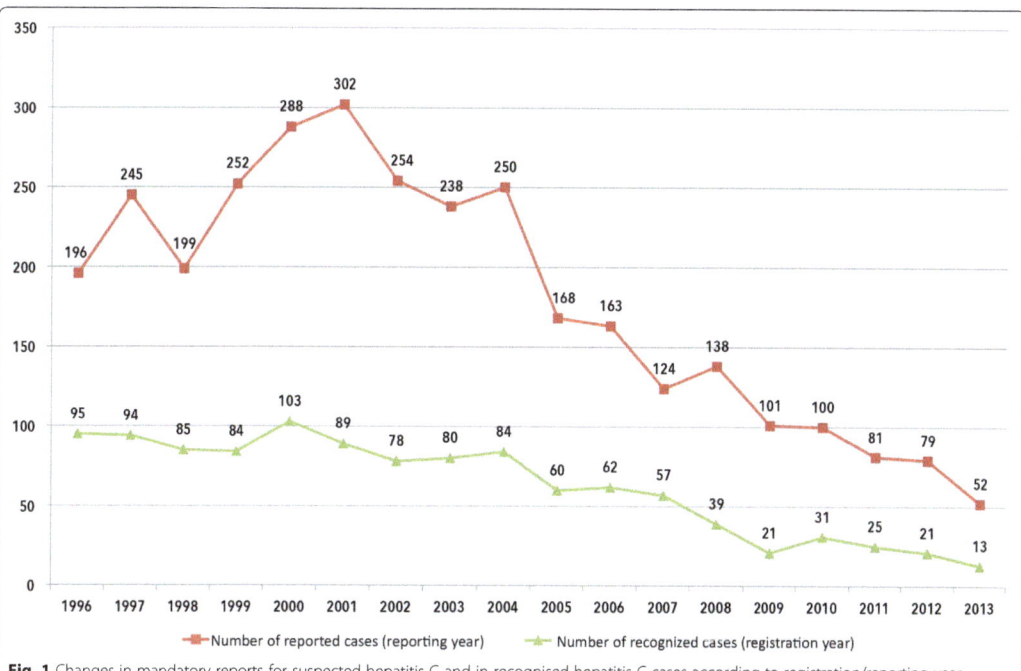

Fig. 1 Changes in mandatory reports for suspected hepatitis C and in recognised hepatitis C cases according to registration/reporting year (1996–2013, BGW data)

Westermann *et al. Journal of Occupational Medicine and Toxicology* (2016) 11:52

in accordance with data protection regulations and with the agreement of the BGW Data Protection Officer. The data was analysed using the statistics software SPSS version 23.

Results

In 1996 to 2013, a total of 3230 reports of suspected cases of occupational HCV diseases were registered with BGW. In the same period, infections were recognised as ODs for 1121 insured parties. Across the study period, the number of reported and recognised cases declined by 73 and 86% respectively (Fig. 1).

Description of the sample (OD cases)

OD reports identified 1121 insured parties with an occupational HCV. Mainly affected were female, older than 40 years of age and employed in hospitals. Over 90% of the insured were engaged in a medical or nursing occupation at the time that they developed the disease (Table 1).

In the period under analysis, 42 deaths were recorded as the result of an OD. Of those, one person was under 30 years of age, 16 (43%) were between 30 and 60 years of age, while 25 (55%) were over the age of 61. The majority of them (67%) were employed in hospitals, with just 21% working in doctor's practices and 11% in residential geriatric care or rehabilitation clinics (no table).

Reduced work ability [RWA]

A total of 70% of insured parties (*n* = 779) had an initial documented RWA in the analysis period from 1996 to 2014. The distribution of the degrees of RWA is shown in Table 1. In 57% of cases, the RWA did not increase during the period of their disease. In just under 40% of cases, there were between two and four changes; only a few had more than five changes. In one case, the RWA changed twelve times.

Of 1121 cases, 75% had no RWA (as of the analysis date of 31 December 2014) (Table 2). These include insured parties who died in the period under analysis (1996 to 2013, *n* = 52). A RWA was established for 779 insured parties over the course of the disease, although a RWA was only in effect for 279 insured parties on the analysis date, showing that 64% of the CHC patients only had a temporary RWA (500 of 779). Breaking down the entire reference period into four intervals shows only minor differences in the RWA grade. Only the 95th percentile and the maximum RWA are higher for cases registered before 2011 than for cases between 2011 and 2013 (40 versus 30% and 100 versus 50%).

Description of changes in expenses

Table 3 lists the payments and number of postings registered. For 98% of the recognised HCV cases, at least one posting was registered during the period of 15 years (*n* =

Table 1 Description of the sample of insured parties with a recognised hepatitis C infection according to sociodemographic characteristics and the degree of reduced work ability (RWA) first established (*n* = 1121)

Characteristics	N	%
Sex, female	838	75
Age (years)[a]		
< 20	17	1
21–40	335	30
41–60	646	58
> 61	123	11
Field of work		
Clinic/hospital	510	46
Doctor's practice	341	30
Geriatric care/nursing	131	12
Outpatient/social welfare services	79	7
Administration	60	5
Occupation		
Physician	195	17
Nurse	473	42
Medical assistant	266	24
Geriatric care assistant	84	8
Medical personnel	31	3
Administration	36	3
Social worker	19	2
Domestic services	17	1
RWA as %[b]		
No RWA	342	30
RWA <20	3	0.4
RWA 20	493	63.2
RWA 30	127	16.3
RWA 40	64	8.2
RWA 50	35	4.5
RWA 60–80	37	4.7
RWA 100	20	2.6
Total	1121	100

[a]Age at the time of registration of the ODs reports
[b]Values relate to RWA as first established

1097). Most postings were attributable to outpatient treatments (40%) and pension disbursements (37%). In the period under analysis, compensation payments came to € 87.9 million, of which just under 60% were attributable to pension payments (€ 51,570,830) and around 15% to expenses for pharmaceuticals and other medicines (€ 12,978,318).

Compensation payments for medical rehabilitation (pharmaceuticals and other medicines), occupational rehabilitation (phased returns, retraining, etc.) and pensions

Publikation 2

Westermann *et al. Journal of Occupational Medicine and Toxicology* (2016) 11:52

Page 5 of 8

Table 2 Documented reduced work ability (RWA) as of the analysis date 31 December 2014 grouped by period of occupational disease (OD) registration

RWA as %	Year of OD registration (grouped)									
	1996 to 2000		2001 to 2005		2006 to 2010		2011 to 2013		Total	
	N	%	N	%	N	%	N	%	N	%
No RWA[a]	357	77	289	74	154	73	42	71	842	75
010	1	0	0	0	1	0	0	0	2	0
020	58	13	53	14	26	12	11	19	148	13
030	15	3	20	5	13	6	4	7	52	5
040	9	2	7	2	5	2	0	0	21	2
050	9	2	5	1	7	3	2	3	23	2
060	4	1	7	2	1	0	0	0	12	1
070	5	1	4	1	0	0	0	0	9	1
080	1	0	1	0	1	0	0	0	3	0
100	2	0	5	1	2	1	0	0	9	1
Total	461	100	391	100	210	100	59	100	1,121	100
P 75	0		20		20		20		0	
P 95	40		40		40		30		40	
Max	100		100		100		50		100	

[a]Total deaths n = 52, of which 42 resulting from occupational disease (1996–2000 n = 18; 2001–2005 n = 14; 2006–2010 n = 8; 2011–2013 n = 2); not resulting from occupational disease (1996–2000 n = 6; 2001–2005 n = 3; 2006–2010 n = 1)

have developed differently over the 15-year period under review (Fig. 2). Annual expenses rose from € 2.6 million to € 6.3 million between 2000 and 2005, remaining at an annual € 6 million between 2005 and 2010 before then rising to € 7.3 million and € 8.3 million in 2012 and 2014 respectively. In all years except 2014, payments for medical rehabilitation accounted for around one third, while expenses for pensions accounted for around two thirds of the costs. In 2014 on the other hand, expenses for medical rehabilitation accounted for around half of expenditure. Pension payments came to € 1.6 million in 2000 and rose continuously to over € 4 million in 2014. Benefits aimed at enabling involvement in working life (occupational rehabilitation) accounted for less than 1% in all years.

Drugs for the treatment of hepatitis C

For the sample of recognised HCV cases, expenses for drugs of € 255,730 in 2000 first rose continuously to around € 1 million and remained at this level until 2010, with the exception of 2007 (Fig. 3). A clear rise in expenses for drugs was recorded for 2012 (to around € 1.7 million) and 2014 (to around € 2.5 million). Relative to

Table 3 Accounting entry descriptions (grouped) according to number of cases, number of postings and expenses for recognised HCV cases – added together from 2000 to 2014; sorted by percentage share of total costs

Entry descriptions	Number of cases	Number of entries (%)	Expenses in	
			€	%s
Pensions	862	69,585 (37)	51,570,830	59
Pharmaceuticals and other medicines from pharmacies	619	9,897 (5)	12,978,318	14
Injury compensation, care allowances and other treatment costs	586	10,397 (6)	8,461,788	10
Inpatient treatment	543	1,669 (1)	5,460,608	6
Outpatient treatment (including treatment costs by physician)	921	74,376 (40)	4,812,063	6
Diagnosis costs	1,050	14,910 (8)	3,576,946	4
Benefits aimed at enabling involvement in working life (occupational rehabilitation)	49	1,310 (1)	730,423	1
Costs for resources	78	345 (0)	206,087	0
Reports	631	4,492 (2)	60,564	0
Total[a]	5,339[b]	186,981 (100)	87,857,627	100

[a]Does not include combined invoices and payments received for rehabilitation (n = 19,445, 9%), [b]Cases may arise in more than one posting description (e.g., costs for treatments, reports and pharmaceuticals)

Publikation 2

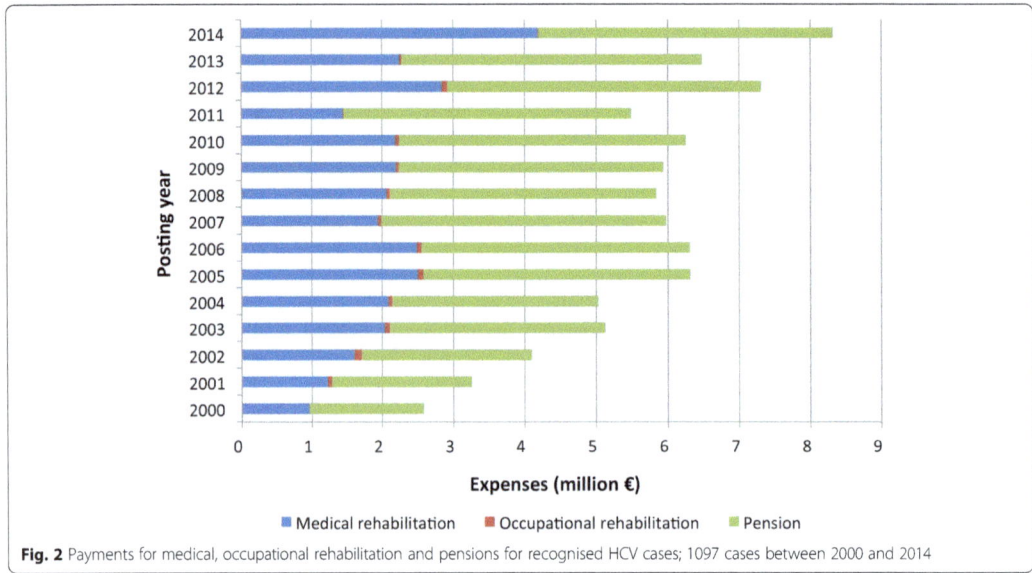

Fig. 2 Payments for medical, occupational rehabilitation and pensions for recognised HCV cases; 1097 cases between 2000 and 2014

the annual costs incurred for the years 2005 to 2010, the increase in costs for drugs was over 70% in 2012 and over 120% in 2014.

Discussion

Among German healthcare personnel workers, both reported and recognized occupational HCV infections decreased over the study period, yet costs associated with HCV increased. The majority of claims was represented by females aged 40 years and older who were employed as nurses in hospitals. The anti-HCV prevalence in the general population in Germany is estimated to be stable at a low level (0.3%) [10]. The number of reported OD cases among healthcare personnel in Germany declined over the

time possibly due to improved blood-borne pathogen handling practices. Guidelines have been issued since 2000 that aim to prevent exposure to blood, for example, from NSI [11]. In the mid-1990s it came to a strong increase in reported ODs, probably in many cases linked to old cases, as a result of increased investigations since the mid-1990s in Germany [12]. In addition, the number of reported and recognized ODs may not reflect the real number of HCV infection cases among healthcare personnel. Needlestick injuries (NSI) are the most frequently reported occupational accidents in healthcare [13]. The results of epidemiological studies indicate that most of HCWs (80%) have been affected by NSI, and many such injuries remain unreported [11].

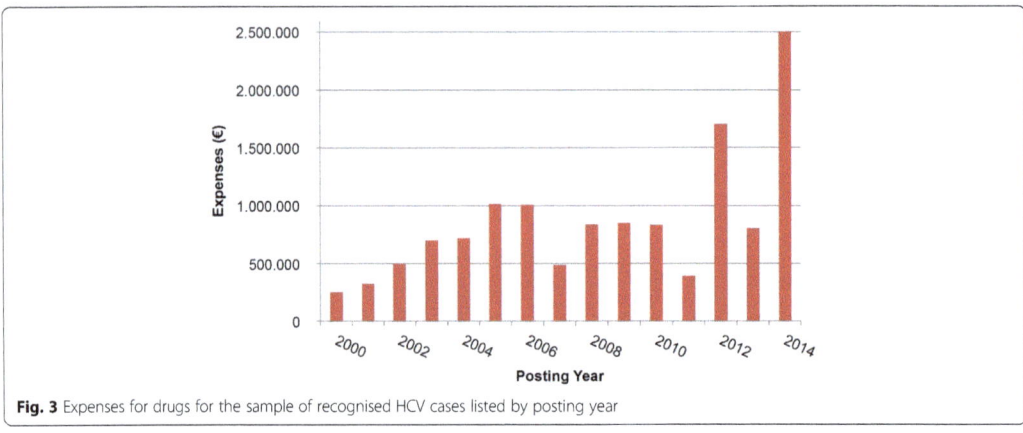

Fig. 3 Expenses for drugs for the sample of recognised HCV cases listed by posting year

Publikation 2

Westermann *et al. Journal of Occupational Medicine and Toxicology* (2016) 11:52

Page 7 of 8

Despite lower OD HCV prevalence, the costs related to occupational exposure have increased. The costs for CHC are largely defined by the rising expenses for pensions. In 2012 to 2014, however, there was a strong rise in each case in costs for drug therapy. This likely associated with expenses for triple combinations of pegylated interferon, ribavirin and one of the two first-generation protease inhibitors, boceprevir and telaprevir in 2012. The rise in expenses in 2014 is probably attributable to the use of new direct antiviral agents (DAAs, second-generation protease inhibitors) for the treatment of HCV infections.

Initial research results on the new DAAs indicate sustainable SVR rates with shorter treatment periods and a tendency for fewer side effects [4]. DAAs initially involve higher expenses, but may reduce long term treatment costs as reported by Nevens et al. [14]. SVR rates are associated with a reduction in CHC-caused (hepatic and extrahepatic) morbidity and mortality [15, 16]. Functional improvements in the cirrhosis were observed through the SVRs, as were sustained successes in the treatment of extrahepatic complications [4, 8]. CHC remains the most frequent indication for liver transplantation [17]. Preoperative treatment to achieve an SVR at the time of transplantation sustainably reduces the risk of the transplanted organ being infected with the HCV [15, 17]. Early identification of an infection is a key factor in enabling the patient to recover as fully as possible. The treatment of patients in less severe stages of the disease using DAA therapy is costly, but is likely to be successful in preventing future advanced liver diseases that are also associated with high expense [6]. Nevens et al. also observed a considerable reduction in the costs in cases where an SVR was achieved in the mild, less pronounced phases of CHC [14]. In the long term, the high costs of this treatment are likely to pay off by allowing early treatment of CHC infections to reduce morbidity and mortality rates. The case figures presented here do not provide a complete picture of the costs for occupation HCV infections in Germany. The BGW database used here only contains OD reports on employees from non-government institutions. Those restrictions that generally apply for secondary data apply to this register data. The data is not clinical in nature, but rather administrative with limited sociodemographic characteristics present. As in table one reported, nurses are the largest represented demographic group among the healthcare professionals with an HCV infection as OD. This data was not corrected for the total population because it was not possible to get the necessary information, with the same corresponding to the age groups presented. Although this lack of data adjustment is an inherent limitation of our study, a positive feature of this data is that it provides a longitudinal perspective, enabling the claiming of insurance benefits as relevant outcome (e.g., in the form of compensation payments) to be observed over a sufficiently long period of time.

Conclusions

For hepatitis C infections as an OD, a considerable increase in costs has been observed, while the number of cases has declined heavily. These costs are explained by the increase in pension payments and, since 2012, by a rise in the costs for drugs. The use of DAA treatments is currently fundamentally changing disease management for CHC patients. The high costs of the treatments might be offset by the potentially considerable benefits. The optimum solution is successful therapy at as early a stage in the disease as possible in order to preserve the health-related quality of life of the insured as fully as possible, thereby also preserving their ability to work. The resultant reduction in concomitant hepatic and extrahepatic diseases will potentially result in lower RWA gradings in the long term among the overall insured population. In the long run, maintaining the ability to work would generate overall cost savings for accident insurers and also for the other social security systems.

Abbreviations
BGW: Berufsgenossenschaft für Gesundheitsdienst und Wohlfahrtspflege; BK-DOK: BGW's occupational disease routine data records; CHC: Chronic hepatitis C; DAA: Direct anti-viral agent; HCV: Viral hepatitis C; OD: Occupational disease; RWA: Reduced work ability; STROSA: A consensus German reporting standard for secondary data analyses; SVR: Sustained virological response; WHO: World health organisation

Acknowledgements
We would like to thank the Rehabilitation Coordination Department (BGW) for their support.

Funding
No special funds were received for this study. However, the Institute for Health Services Research in Dermatology and Nursing of the University Medical Centre Hamburg-Eppendorf (UKE) receives an unrestricted fund from the Institution for Statutory Accident Insurance and Prevention in the Health and Welfare services (BGW) on an annual basis to maintain the working group at the UKE. The funds are provided by a non-profit organization that is part of the social security system in Germany. The funder had no role in study design, data collection and analysis, decision to publish, or preparation of the manuscript.

Availability of data and materials
The original data are property of the Institution for Statutory Accident Insurance and Prevention in the Health and Welfare Services (BGW). The aggregated data as they were provided by the insurance are available upon request by the head of the department Prof. Dr. Albert Nienhaus (a.nienhaus@uke.de).

Authors' contributions
MD, CW and AN developed the study design. DW and MD conducted the data analysis. The interpretation of the data was made by MD, DW, CW and AN. CW wrote the manuscript, with significant contribution from the other authors. Uncertainties were discussed between the authors regularly. AN revised the manuscript critically for important intellectual content and gave final approval for the version to be published. All authors read and approved the final manuscript.

Competing interests
The authors declare that they have no competing interests.

Consent for publication
All authors read and approved the final manuscript and gave approval for publication.

Publikation 2

Westermann *et al. Journal of Occupational Medicine and Toxicology* (2016) 11:52

Page 8 of 8

Ethics approval and consent to participate

The study was not submitted to an ethic commission as only anonym routine data of an insurance were used and no personal data were collected and no medical test was performed in the scope of the study. However, the study was accepted by the data protection board of the insurance which provided the data. In accordance with the Professional Code for Physicians in Hamburg (Art. 15, 1., Status of 10.03.2014) and the Chamber Legislation for Medical Professions in the Federal State of Hamburg (HmbKGH) it is only necessary to obtain advice on questions of professional ethics and professional conduct from an Ethics Committee if data which can be traced to a particular individual is being used in a research project.

Author details

[1]University Medical Center Hamburg-Eppendorf (UKE), Center of Excellence for Health Services Research in Nursing (CVcare), Hamburg, Germany. [2]Institution for Statutory Accident Insurance and Prevention in the Health and Welfare Services (BGW), Department of Prevention and Rehabilitation Principles (GPR), Hamburg, Germany.

Received: 9 September 2016 Accepted: 16 November 2016
Published online: 24 November 2016

References

1. Askarian M, Yadollahi M, Kuochak F, Danaei M, Vakili V, Momeni M. Precautions for health care workers to avoid hepatitis B and C virus infection. Int J Occup Environ Med. 2011;2:191–8.
2. Westermann C, Peters C, Lisiak B, Lamberti M, Nienhaus A. The prevalence of hepatitis C among healthcare workers: a systematic review and meta-analysis. Occup Environ Med. 2015;72:880–8.
3. WHO. WHO Guidelines Approved by the Guidelines Review Committee. Geneva: Guidelines for the Screening Care and Treatment of Persons with Chronic Hepatitis C Infection: Updated Version. 2016. (http://www.ncbi.nlm.nih.gov/pubmed/27227200. Accessed 14 Jun 2016).
4. Sarrazin C, Berg TP, Buggisch MM, Dollinger H, Hinrichsen H, Hofer DH, et al. Aktuelle Empfehlung zur Therapie der chronischen Hepatitis C S3 guideline hepatitis C addendum. Z Gastroenterol. 2015;53:320–34.
5. WHO. Hepatitis C - Fact sheet Geneva: N°164. 2014. (http://www.who.int/mediacentre/factsheets/fs164/en/. Accessed 4 Feb 2016).
6. Gordon SC, Pockros PJ, Terrault NA, Hoop RS, Buikema A, Nerenz D, et al. Impact of disease severity on healthcare costs in patients with chronic hepatitis C (CHC) virus infection. Hepatol (Baltimore, Md). 2012;56:1651–60.
7. Younossi ZM, Singer ME, Mir HM, Henry L, Hunt S. Impact of interferon free regimens on clinical and cost outcomes for chronic hepatitis C genotype 1 patients. J Hepatol. 2014;60:530–7.
8. Westbrook RH, Dusheiko G. Natural history of hepatitis C. J Hepatol. 2014;61 Suppl 1:58–68.
9. Swart E, Bitzer EM, Gothe H, Harling M, Hoffmann F, Horenkamp-Sonntag D, et al. A consensus German reporting standard for secondary data analyses, version 2 (STROSA-STandardisierte BerichtsROutine fur SekundardatenAnalysen). Gesundheitswesen (Bundesverband der Arzte des Offentlichen Gesundheitsdienstes (Germany). 2016;78(SO1):e145–260.
10. Poethko-Muller C, Zimmermann R, Hamouda O, Faber M, Stark K, Ross RS, et al. Epidemiology of hepatitis a, B, and C among adults in Germany: results of the German health interview and examination survey for adults (DEGS1). Bundesgesundheitsblatt, Gesundheitsforschung, Gesundheitsschutz. 2013; 56(5–6):707–15.
11. Elseviers MM, Arias-Guillen M, Gorke A, Arens HJ. Sharps injuries amongst healthcare workers: review of incidence, transmissions and costs. J Ren Care. 2014;40(3):150–6.
12. Dulon ML B, Wendeler D, Nienhaus A. Occupational infectious diseases in healthcare workers 2014. Data from the institution for statutory accident insurance and prevention in the health and welfare services. Zentralbl Arbeitsmed Arbeitsschutz Ergon. 2015;65:210–6.
13. Nienhaus A, Kesavachandran C, Wendeler D, Haamann F, Dulon M. Infectious diseases in healthcare workers - an analysis of the standardised data set of a German compensation board. J Occup Med Toxicol. 2012;7(1):8.
14. Nevens F, Colle I, Michielsen P, Robaeys G, Moreno C, Caekelbergh K, et al. Resource use and cost of hepatitis C-related care. Eur J Gastroenterol Hepatol. 2012;24:1191–8.
15. Gonzalez-Grande R, Jimenez-Perez M, Gonzalez Arjona C, Mostazo TJ. New approaches in the treatment of hepatitis C. World J Gastroenterol. 2016;22:1421–32.
16. Tada T, Kumada T, Toyoda H, Kiriyama S, Tanikawa M, Hisanaga Y, et al. Viral eradication reduces all-cause mortality in patients with chronic hepatitis C virus infection: a propensity score analysis. Liver Int. 2016;36(6):817–26.
17. Fagiuoli S, Ravasio R, Luca MG, Baldan A, Pecere S, Vitale A, et al. Management of hepatitis C infection before and after liver transplantation. World J Gastroenterol. 2015;21:4447–56.

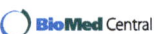

Westermann *et al. Journal of Occupational Medicine and Toxicology* (2018) 13:16
https://doi.org/10.1186/s12995-018-0197-6

Journal of Occupational
Medicine and Toxicology

RESEARCH

Open Access

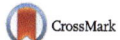

Hepatitis C in healthcare personnel: secondary data analysis of therapies with direct-acting antiviral agents

Claudia Westermann[1*] ⓘ, Dana Wendeler[2] and Albert Nienhaus[1,2]

Abstract

Background: Hepatitis C Virus (HCV) infections are blood-borne, generally chronic and are associated with increased morbidity and mortality. The aim of this study is to describe the results of therapies with direct-acting antiviral agents (DAAs) in healthcare personnel.

Methods: Secondary data analysis using data from the Statutory Accident Insurance of the Health and Welfare Service. The study surveyed DAA therapies administered to insured parties (healthcare personnel with an HCV infection recognised as an occupational disease) in Germany between 01/01/2014 and 30/11/2016. The end points were results of monitorings carried out twelve weeks after the end of treatment (SVR12), side effects and the results of the assessment of reduced work ability after treatment. Multivariate logistic regression models were constructed to model SVR12.

Results: The study population ($n = 180$) comprised 74% women, 90% of the participants had an HCV genotype 1 infection. Two-thirds had fibrosis or cirrhosis and were treatment experienced. The most common combined therapy was ledipasvir and sofosbuvir (49%). A DAA therapy with ribavirin was administered in 20% of cases, with (pegylated) interferon and ribavirin used in 2% of cases. The majority of therapies were completed without any side effects. The overall SVR12 rate was 94%. Significant independent predictor of decrease odds of SVR12 was liver cirrhosis. Positive effects on the healthcare personnel's work ability were observed after successful therapy.

Conclusion: High SVR12 rates were achieved in the sample population, with positive effects on their work ability. Early HCV therapy seems reasonable due to the increased chance of successful treatment of the infection.

Keywords: Hepatitis C virus, Occupational exposure, Blood-borne infections, Healthcare personnel, Direct-acting antiviral agents

Background

The hepatitis C virus (HCV) is one of the most common infectious diseases in the world and develops into a chronic infection in up to 85% of cases. According to data from the World Health Organisation (WHO), approx. 71 million people globally have a chronic hepatitis C (CHC) infection [1, 2]. CHC is associated with higher morbidity and higher mortality [2, 3]. The use of direct-acting antiviral agents (DAAs) is currently leading to a major shift in the management of chronic HCV infections. DAAs open up the possibility for efficient oral therapy regimens with fewer side effects for patients with or without treatment experience. As recent studies have shown, interferon-free DAA treatments have achieved substantial sustained virological response rates (SVRs) of over 90% [4, 5]. For CHC infections, treatment success is achieved when the HCV virus's RNA can no longer be detected in the blood (SVR), generally twelve weeks after the end of treatment [6, 7]. SVRs are associated with lowering morbidity and mortality caused by CHC [8, 9].

* Correspondence: c.westermann@uke.de
[1]Competence Centre for Epidemiology and Health Services Research for Healthcare Professionals (CVcare), Institute for Health Services Research in Dermatology and Nursing (IVDP), University Medical Centre Hamburg-Eppendorf (UKE), Martinistr. 52, 20146 Hamburg, Germany
Full list of author information is available at the end of the article

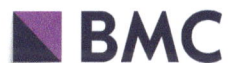

Publikation 3

Westermann *et al. Journal of Occupational Medicine and Toxicology* (2018) 13:16   Page 2 of 8

Healthcare personnel (HP) have contact with infected patients as part of their work. Injuries caused by sharp or pointed objects are some of the most commonly reported workplace accidents [10]. In Germany, reports detailing a reasonable suspicion of occupational illness are submitted to the statutory accident insurance carriers. Despite being on the decrease, Hepatitis C is still one of the most common infections leading to the recognition of an occupational illness among German HP. It is also the most common reason for newly approved retirement on the grounds of occupational disease [11]. Data analysis of an accident insurer shows that despite the number of cases has declined, the costs of HCV infection as an occupational disease (OD) have been significantly increasing over the past 15 years. These costs are the result of the increase in compensation payments for retirement on the grounds of OD and, since 2012, as a result of an increase in the cost of the drugs used to treat the infection [12]. The high costs of DAA therapies are offset by the potentially considerable benefits. The aim of this study is to investigate the treatment results of the DAA therapies in HP.

Methods

Analysis of the DAA therapies using data from the Statutory Accident Insurance of the Health and Welfare Service (Berufsgenossenschaft für Gesundheitsdienst und Wohlfahrtspflege, BGW). This analysis was carried out in line with the Consensus German Reporting Standard for Secondary Data Analyses (STROSA) [13]. When applying for DAA therapy for a HP with an occupational CHC infection, the BGW collects data (using a standardised input mask (Excel table)) about the course of treatment for the purposes of conducting an analysis. For quality assurance purposes, this process was discussed and aided by the BGW's Occupational Diseases working group. Following data was anonymised extracted from doctors' letters and test results in the insured party's medical files: genotype, reduced work ability (RWA) grading, treatments used, treatment status (naive/experienced), cirrhosis (yes/no), start and end of treatment (duration), treatment result (RNA evidence), side effects, and assessment of the RWA after DAA therapy. The analysis included data from insured individuals who completed DAA therapy between 01/01/2014 and 30/11/2016 and for whom treatment results were available twelve weeks after the end of therapy. In cases of treatment failure directly following the end of therapy, if there was no data available at twelve weeks after the end of treatment, it was also assumed that treatment had failed. Evidence of virus RNA twelve weeks after the end of treatment following previous ETR (end-of-treatment sustained virological response) was considered a relapse. The end points investigated were treatment success

twelve weeks after the end of treatment (SVR12), side effects and the results of assessment of the RWA after the conclusion of DAA therapy.

Determination of RWA in occupational disease procedures

Statutory accident insurance is one of the pillars of German social insurance. On the basis of the 7th German Social Security Code (Siebtes Buch, Sozialgesetzbuch, SGB VII), every employer is legally obliged to insure employees against accidents at work. The sponsorship of statutory accident insurance, the group of insured persons and the procedure in the event of a claim as well as the benefits in the event of an insured event are regulated in this code of law. The essential benefit for insured persons who get injured at the workplace following an accident or who suffer an occupational disease is the entitlement to compensation if their performance and thus their ability to work cannot be fully restored. This entitlement for the injured person's pension is dependent on the assessment of the RWA and the extent to which the reduction in the physical and mental capacity of an insured person restricts their work opportunities. In the event of a complete loss of working ability (100%), a full pension is paid, which amounts to two thirds of the annual earnings before the occupational disease. In the case of a partial RWA, a partial pension corresponding to the degree of RWA is paid. The entitlement starts with a RWA of at least 20%. For claimants suffering HCV, the RWA is determined by the fibrosis stage and the degree of inflammatory activity of the disease. The initial assessment requires a detailed anamnesis, the clinical status and an abdominal sonography as well as a sufficient laboratory program with clinical-chemical, virological and immunoserological parameters. A reliable differential diagnostic and functional assessment of the liver situation needs to be ensured. Further assessment criteria are the probable duration and the course of the disease and the associated statement on the prognosis. A RWA of 20% should be granted when the CHC infection is accompanied with an increased concentration of the liver enzymes but not with a fibrosis of the liver, whereas a RWA of 50 to 100% should be granted when a cirrhosis is present. However, the grading is performed individually and personal circumstances like fatigue or depression should also be considered. The grading is performed by the case manager of the insurance with the support of a physician. The RWA determines the amount of the pension to be paid, even over the period of working life.

Statistical analysis

Univariate comparisons were made to describe the correlations between treatment success (SVR12) and the categorical variables treatment status (naive/experienced),

Publikation 3

Westermann *et al. Journal of Occupational Medicine and Toxicology* (2018) 13:16   Page 3 of 8

cirrhosis (yes/no), RWA (≤50%/> 50%) and gender. The significance of the correlations was tested using the Fisher's exact test. Pearson's correlation coefficient was calculated to measure the statistical association between age and RWA. Multivariate logistic regression models were constructed to model SVR12. Models included cirrhosis, prior treatment, gender, and age (as a continuous variable). Nagelkerke's R-squared was calculated and used to derive Cohen's effect size [14]. Using the measure according to Cohen, an f-value of 0.10 equates to a small effect, an f-value of 0.25 to a medium effect and an f-value of 0.40 to a large effect. For all comparisons, a p-Value < 0.05 was considered statistically significant. Data analysis was done using IBM SPSS Statistics version 23.

Results

During the analysis period, a DAA therapy was administered to 180 HP and the SVR was determined twelve weeks after the end of treatment.

Description of the sample (Table 1)

The mean age of the insured individuals was 62 years. For the period under analysis, 60% were under the statutory retirement age of 65 years. The sample population comprised 74% women. The most common type of infection among the sample was HCV genotype 1 (91%), with individual cases caused by viruses of genotypes 2, 3 or 4. No co-morbidities with Hepatitis B or HIV infections were documented. There were histological indications in 76% of the participants (fibrosis 43%; compensated or decompensated cirrhosis 24 and 9%, respectively) before the DAA therapy started and 72% had already experienced a prior treatment. More than 90% of the insured individuals had a RWA, approximately a third had a RWA of more than 50%.

DAA-regimens and side effects (Table 2)

The most common treatment was a combination therapy of ledipasvir (LDV) and sofosbuvir (SOF) ($n = 88/49\%$). A DAA therapy with ribavirin (RBV) was administered in 36 cases (20%), and (pegylated) interferon (PEG-IFN) and RBV were used in four cases (2%). Treatment duration was between eight and 24 weeks, with the majority lasting twelve weeks (71%). For 67% of insured individuals, the treatment was not associated with any side effects. The most common side effect was a combination of mild symptoms such as headaches, nausea and sleep disorders and/or fatigue (26%). 4% of the sample population suffered from skin reactions (pruritus to generalised skin rash, phototoxic reactions), and there were individual cases of decrease in haemoglobin, feelings of anxiety or depression and isolated gastrointestinal disorders. Side effects not linked to the DAA therapy, but seen as symptoms of an

Table 1 Baseline characteristics ($n = 180$)

Characteristic (missing values n/%)	Valid values	
	n	%
Gender		
Women	133	74
Men	47	26
Age		
Mean (SD)	62 (10)	
Median/Minimum/Maximum	62/21/88	
Age group		
30–39	4	2
40–49	12	7
50–59	50	28
60–64	42	23
≥ 65[a]	72	40
Genotype (11/6)		
1 sub-type not recognised	15	9
1a	50	29
1b	88	52
2	6	4
3	7	4
3a	2	1
4	1	< 1
RWA % (5/3)		
0 < 20	12	7
20	59	34
30–40	46	26
50–60	35	20
70–80	11	6
90–100	12	7
Stage of liver disease (28/16)		
No findings	37	24
Fibrosis	65	43
Compensated cirrhosis	37	24
Decompensated cirrhosis	13	9
Therapy status (21/12)		
Naive	45	28
Experienced	114	72

[a]statutory retirement age; *RWA* reduced work ability, *SD* standard deviation

advanced CHC infection were summarised as other side effects (bleeding of the oesophageal varices, incipient hepatorenal syndrome). The observed side effects of a decrease in haemoglobin ($n = 2$) occurred in DAA therapy (LDV/SOF) combined with RBV in priory treated patients with liver cirrhosis. These therapies were conducted for twelve or 24 weeks and led to SVR12 in the insured individuals. Anxiety and depression were observed in

Westermann *et al. Journal of Occupational Medicine and Toxicology* (2018) 13:16

Table 2 DAA treatment regimens and results (n = 180)

Characteristic (missing values n/%)	Valid values	
	n	%
Therapies total (2/1)	178	
LDV, SOF	88	49
SOF, DCV	29	16
LDV, SOF, RBV	17	10
SOF, SMV	11	6
DSV, OBV, PTV, RTV, RBV	11	6
DSV, OBV, PTV, RTV	9	5
SOF, RBV	7	4
SOF, RBV, PEG-IFN	3	2
DCV, SOF, RBV	1	< 1
SOF, SMV, RBV	1	< 1
PEG-IFN, TVR, RBV	1	< 1
Therapy result		
Directly after therapy (1/< 1)	179	
ETR	173	97
Remission	6	3
Twelve weeks after therapy	180	
SVR12	170	94
Remission/viral load unchanged	6	> 2
Relapse	4	> 3
Side effects (13/7)	167	
None	110	66
Headaches, nausea, sleep disorder	43	26
Skin reactions	6	4
Anaemia	2	> 1
Depression, anxiety	2	> 1
Gastrointestinal disorders	2	> 1
Other[a]	2	> 1

[a]Manifestation of advanced infection (hepatorenal syndrome n = 1, bleeding of oesophageal varices n = 1); *DAA* direct-acting antiviral agents, *LDV* ledipasvir, *SOF* sofosbuvir, *DCV* daclatasvir, *RBV* ribavirin, *RTV* ritonavir, *SMV* simeprevir, *DSV* dasabuvir, *OBV* ombitasvir, *PTV* paritaprevir, *PEG-IFN* pegylated interferon, *TVR* telaprevir, *ETR* end-of-treatment response, *SVR12* sustained virologic response twelve weeks after therapy

patients with treatment experience and without liver cirrhosis (n = 2) receiving DAA therapies in combination with ribavirin or PEG-IFN (SOF/RBV/PEG-IFN; dasabuvir (DSV)/ombitasvir (OBV)/paritaprevir (PTV)/ ritonavir (RTV)/RBV). These were completed after the standard twelve weeks and led to SVR12 in the insured individuals.

Treatment results and summary statistics

The ETR rate was 97% and the SVR12 rate was 94% (Table 2). Virus RNA could still be detected in six individuals directly after the end of treatment. At the results monitoring twelve weeks after the end of treatment, six

patients showed no change or a reduction in viral load, while four patients had a relapse (Additional file 1: Table S1). The results of univariate and logistic regression analysis regarding treatment response (SVR12) are described in Table 3. Prior experience of treatment resulted in no significant difference in terms of SVR12 (naive n = 45/experienced n = 114: SVR12 98% vs 94%, p = 0.44), while there was a statistically significant difference with regard to cirrhosis status. For individuals without cirrhosis (n = 102), the treatment was statistically significant more likely to be successful than for patients with diagnosed cirrhosis (n = 50) (SVR12 98% vs 86%, p = 0.006). For insured individuals with a RWA grading of ≤50% (n = 139), the DAA treatment was also statistically significant more likely to be successful than for patients with a higher RWA grading (n = 36) (SVR12 97% vs 86%, p = 0.019). It was somewhat more likely for women (n = 133) to reach SVR12 after therapy than men (n = 47) (SVR12 96% vs 89%, p = 0.130). The multivariate regression showed that cirrhosis was a statistically significant independent predictor of decrease odds of SVR12. Participants with cirrhosis were 10 percentage points less likely to reach SVR12 in comparison to patients without cirrhosis. This resulted in an adjusted OR of 0.098 (95% CI 0.01–0.75; p = 0.03). With an increase in age, there was also an increase in the probability of achieving SVR12 (OR 1.11; 95% CI 1.01–1.23, p = 0.04). The variables of prior treatment (OR 0.42; 95% CI 0.05–3.92; p = 0.42) and gender (OR 0.41; 95% CI 0.08–2.18; p = 0.3) showed no statistically significant correlation with the end-point SVR12 in the multivariate analysis. Nagelkerke's R-squared was 0.24, which corresponds to an f-value of 0.56, which Cohen classifies as a large effect size. The liver enzyme laboratory values (GOT, GPT, γGT) for 102 insured individuals at twelve weeks after the end of treatment were available at the time of the evaluation. For 90 (88%) of the individuals, the liver enzymes were in the normal range twelve weeks after the DAA therapy.

Evaluation of RWA after DAA therapy

Evaluation of RWA after DAA therapy was done for 115 (64%) of the insured individuals, on average nine months after the end of treatment. The RWA was adjusted for 87 (76%) of the insured individuals. The RWA determined before treatment lapsed for 56 individuals, 25 individuals had a decrease in the RWA after the evaluation and six increased their RWA (Table 4). Reasons for an increased RWA included liver transplant after successful DAA therapy, bleeding of the oesophageal varices and incipient hepatorenal syndrome. The correlation between age and RWA was low (r = 0.16, p = 0.04).

Westermann *et al. Journal of Occupational Medicine and Toxicology* (2018) 13:16

Table 3 Summary of univariate and logistic regression analysis for variables regarding treatment response SVR12 (n = 180)

Univariate analysis

Variable	Missing values	n total	% SVR12 rates	OR (95% CI)	p-value
Cirrhosis (no/yes)	28	152 (102/50)	98% versus 86%	0.12 (0.03–0.62)	< 0.01
Treatment (naive/experienced)	21	159 (45/114)	97.8% versus 93.9%	0.35 (0.04–2.90)	NS
RWA (≤50%/> 50%)	5	175 (139/36)	97.1% versus 86.1%	0.18 (0.05–0.72)	< 0.05
Gender (women/men)	0	180 (133/47)	96.2% versus 87.5%	0.32 (0.09–1.19)	NS

Multivariate logistical regression model with SVR12 as end point

Variable	Missing values	n total	OR (95% CI)	p-value	R^2
Cirrhosis (no/yes)	34	146 (98/48)	0.098 (0.01–0.75)	< 0.05	0.242
Treatment (naive/experienced)	34	146 (42/104)	0.42 (0.05–3.92)	NS	
Gender (women/men)	34	146 (112/34)	0.41 (0.08–2.18)	NS	
Age[a]	34	146	1.11 (1.01–1.23)	< 0.05	

SVR12 sustained virologic response twelve weeks after therapy, *RWA* reduced work ability; Dependent variables - the first category is established as a reference;
[a]as a continuous variable; OR (odds ratio) for the primary end point of SVR12; *NS* non-significant

Discussion

Patients with and without experience of treatment who have a CHC infection achieved high SVR12 (94%) rates in the observed sample. Cirrhosis status (OR 0.098; 95% CI 0.01–0.75; p = 0.03) and age (OR 1.11; 95% CI 1.01–1.23; p = 0.04) had a significant correlation with treatment success. Significant independent predictor of decrease odds of SVR12 was liver cirrhosis. Even though, the correlation between age and SVR12 was statistically significant, advanced age is no barrier to DAA therapy. SVRs are associated with reducing morbidity and mortality resulting from a CHC infection, irrespective of individual cirrhosis status. They are also associated with an improvement in health-related quality of life [8, 9, 15, 16]. In the study population, positive effects on the patients' RWA were observed on average nine months after successful completion of therapy. An evaluation was carried out in 64% of the insured individuals after DAA therapy, showing an improvement in work ability for more than 70% of those being analysed. Hence we assume that pension payments will decrease as well.

In a study with patients with a genotype 1 HCV infection, Backus et al. [17] investigated predictors of achieving SVR (at least ten weeks after the end of treatment) to determine the efficacy of LDV/SOF ± RBV and OBV/PTV/RTV/DSV ± RBV. The variables included in the multivariate analysis were treatment status (naive/experienced), ethnic background, body mass index (BMI), cirrhosis status (FIB-4 > 3.25), age and gender. SVR rates of 94% were achieved in the patient collective (average age: 61, 96% male, 23% with experience of treatment, 30% with cirrhosis). Cirrhosis status (OR 0.60; 95% CI 0–49–0.72, p = 0.001), having an African-American background (OR 0.71; 95% CI 0.59–0.86, p = 0.001) and a BMI of ≥30 kg/m^2 (OR 0.73, 95% CI 0.60–0.89, p = 0.002) had a significant correlation with achieving SVR. In another study, no significant differences were found between treatment naive patients with and without cirrhosis in terms of SVR12 (97.9% vs 96.2%) [18]. Overall, the authors reported that no relapses were observed in patients once they had achieved SVR12. According to Zeuzem [19], the lack of evidence of HCV

Table 4 Reduced work ability before and after DAA therapy (n = 115)

RWA as %		After DAA therapy						Overall	
Before DAA therapy		0	20	30–40	50–60	70–80	90–100	n	%
	0	6	0	0	0	0	0	6	5.2
	20	38	7	1	0	0	0	46	40
	30–40	15	4	7	1	0	0	27	23.5
	50–60	2	2	10	6	0	0	20	17.4
	70–80	1	0	1	0	4	3	9	7.8
	90–100	0	0	0	0	4	3	7	6.1
Overall	n	62	13	19	7	8	6	115	
	%	53.9	11.3	16.5	6.1	7	5.2	100	100

RWA reduced work ability, *DAA* direct-acting antiviral agents

Westermann et al. Journal of Occupational Medicine and Toxicology (2018) 13:16

RNA twelve weeks after the end of DAA therapy signifies a permanent eradication of the virus. Relapses after this point are rare and generally take the form of a reinfection [19]. The most common DAA combination therapy administered in the observed sample was LDV/SOF (49%) and, according to Zimmermann et al. [20], was also the most commonly administered among patients with statutory health insurance in Germany (64%) in 2015. The frequency of the combination of DAA treatments with RBV was not quantified in that particular study. The authors stated a decrease in prescriptions of monthly PEG-IFN therapy regimes from around 2700 in January 2014 to around 650 in December 2015. In this study, a DAA therapy with RBV was administered in 36 cases (20%), and the combination with PEG-IFN and RBV was used in four cases (2%). Treatment was generally administered for twelve weeks (67%). Comparable treatment periods were also observed in the German Hepatitis Cohort (GECCO) [20]. The most commonly described side effects in our study, which were mainly described as mild, were nausea, headaches and sleep disorders, and were also listed by Zeuzem [19] for therapies with SOF and simeprevir (SMV). According to the author, photosensitivity reactions have also been observed during treatment using SMV. These were also observed in our study during combination treatment with SMV, without any consequences for the course of treatment. Decreased haemoglobin was observed in two DAA treatments with LDV/SOF in combination with RBV. The occurrence of haemolytic anaemia during treatment with RBV has been documented in the literature. The therapies were administered successfully (SVR12). In addition, side effects such as anxiety and depression were observed in two individuals with DAA treatments in combination with RBV or PEG-IFN (SOF/RBV/PEG-IFN, DSV/OBV/PTV/RTV/RBV). The treatments were successfully completed (SVR12). The occurrence of depression has been described in the literature both for PEG-IFN and RBV, and particularly when administered as a combination therapy [21, 22].

Cost effectiveness models analysed in the review by Nuno Solinis et al. [15] show that interferon-free DAA therapies are more cost effective than previous interferon-based therapies. The models also showed that early treatment is more cost-effective than therapy in later stages of the disease.

Data analyses showed an increase of costs associated with HCV as an OD in the period from 2000 to 2014 [12]. Despite lower OD HCV prevalence, the cost related to occupational exposure have increased in this period. About of € 87.9 million were spend by the statutory accident insurance for HCV as OD ($n = 1.121$), of which 60% were attributable to pension payments and around

15% to expenses for pharmaceuticals and other medicines. The cost of CHC are largely defined by the rising expenses for pensions due to increase in RWA. However, there was a strong rise in cost of drug therapy in 2012 to 2014 from € 1.7 to € 2.7 million. In 2015, the cost of antiviral drugs for CHC as OD increased to approximately € 11.9 million [23]. As reported by Zimmermann et al. [20], in 2014 about € 664 million were spent on HCV antivirals by the German statutory health insurance (SHI) and approximately € 1.3 billion in 2015. In Germany, more than 70 million persons are insured by the SHI, which represents about 85% of the German population. DAAs initially involve higher expenses, but as an effective treatment they may reduce long term treatment costs. Although the therapy success is convincing, and in Germany anyone with CHC has general access to DAA therapy, prescriptions have been showing a downward trend among patients with statutory health insurance since the end of 2015 [20]. Some possible reasons listed are insecurities regarding the authorisation of treatments and a lack of clarity in the reimbursement system. As a result of the unspecific course of the disease, researchers assume that around 100,000 people in Germany may have an HCV infection and not know about it [24, 25]. According to the WHO, less than 5% of people with chronic hepatitis worldwide (hepatitis B and C) are aware of their status [26]. The lack of compulsory screening strategies for at-risk groups (e.g. HP, intravenous drug users (IVD), men who have sex with men (MSM) and migrants from countries with high prevalence rates) has been criticised internationally [21, 25, 26]. The implementation of screening strategies to identify infected individuals and to interrupt the channels of infection is a major step in the prevention of the disease [24, 25]. There is no vaccine against HCV infection and a successfully treated infection does not offer protection against reinfection [19, 27]. To prevent reinfections (i.e. from needle-stick injuries) it is advisable to include employees with DAA therapy into regular check-up schemes.

The case figures presented here do not provide a complete picture for occupational HCV infections. The BGW only records notifications of occupational illness from employees of non-government institutions. This evaluation is based on register data with specific sociodemographic information, the data is not clinical in nature and not always complete (e.g. missing's in stage of liver disease (15.6%) and treatment experience (11.7%)). Information about co-infections with HBV or HIV could not be evaluated from this database in a statistically valid way because it has not been requested in a standardised form. However, we assume that there is a lower likelihood of co-infection with HBV or HIV because the individuals in the study were HP. These employees have

Westermann *et al. Journal of Occupational Medicine and Toxicology* (2018) 13:16

regular check-ups from occupational healthcare practitioners, which include checking their HBV vaccination status. Three quarters of the sample size in the study are female. Men are more commonly affected by HCV infections than women. Men are more often in at-risk groups, such as the IVD and MSM groups, and are more often co-infected with HIV [25, 26]. Interim results from the GECCO study confirm that men are significantly more likely to have an HCV/HIV co-infection than women [4].

Only the occupational acquired HCV as insured event was taken into consideration in this study. We do not have information on co-morbidities not related to the CHC infection. If the working ability is reduced by several insured events, the RWA is determined separately for each insured event. As these co-morbidities are not considered when grading the RWA for CHC the confounding effect should be minor. We expected that with increasing age the RWA would also rise. However, we observed only a low positive correlation between age and RWA ($r = 0.16$, $p = 0.03$).

Our report is based on the experience of a major German statutory accident insurance with the treatment of Hep C carriers in HP with new antiviral drugs. It is a great achievement that HP with a CHC and failed treatments in the past can be successfully treated. The major outcome is the high therapeutic success (SVR12 94%), although the majority of insures had liver disease. Even if not all of them are still in employment and actively working as HP, a decrease in RWA signifies a reduction in individual disease burden and in pension's payments.

Conclusions

Patients with and without experience of treatment who have a CHC infection achieved high SVR rates in the observed sample. Early treatment is preferable in order to keep the individual disease burden as low as possible. It appears that early treatment is also indicated for cost reasons, e.g. as a result of the influence of cirrhosis on treatment success. DAA therapies make it possible to eradicate the HCV viruses, thus enabling early recovery from the chronic infection. SVRs are associated with substantial reductions in the individual disease burden and with the patient maintaining their ability to work. Over the long term, this will probably lead to cost savings for statutory accident insurers and also for other social security systems. However, we require long-term experiences with DAA therapies in order to be able to reliably interpret the results. Successful completion of treatment does not provide protection from reinfection. HCV screening programmes for at-risk groups are therefore essential, even after successful treatment.

Additional file

Additional file 1: Table S1. Characteristics according to treatment response without ETR and/or SVR12. (DOCX 14 kb)

Abbreviations
BGW: Berufsgenossenschaft für Gesundheitsdienst und Wohlfahrtspflege; CHC: Chronic hepatitis C; DAA: Direct-acting antiviral agent; DSV: Dasabuvir; ETR: End-of-treatment sustained virological response rate; GECCO: German Hepatitis Cohort; HBV: Viral hepatitis B; HCV: Viral hepatitis C; HIV: Human immunodeficiency virus; HP: Healthcare personnel; IVD: Intravenous drug users; LDV: Ledipasvir; MSM: Men who have sex with men; OBV: Ombitasvir; OD: Occupational disease; PEG-IFN: Pegylated interferon; PTV: Paritaprevir; RBV: Ribavirin; RNA: Ribonucleic acid; RTV: Ritonavir; RWA: Reduced work ability; SOF: Sofosbuvir; STROSA: A Consensus German Reporting Standard for Secondary Data Analyses; SVR: Sustained virological response rate; WHO: World Health Organisation

Acknowledgements
We would like to thank the Occupational Diseases working group (BGW) for their support.

Funding
No special funds were received for this study. However, the Institute for Health Services Research in Dermatology and Nursing of the University Medical Centre Hamburg-Eppendorf (UKE) receives an unrestricted fund from the Institution for Statutory Accident Insurance and Prevention in the Health and Welfare services (BGW) on an annual basis to maintain the working group at the UKE. The funds are provided by a non-profit organization that is part of the social security system in Germany. The funder had no role in study design, data collection and analysis, decision to publish, or preparation of the manuscript.

Availability of data and materials
The original data are property of the Institution for Statutory Accident Insurance and Prevention in the Health and Welfare Services (BGW). The aggregated data as they were provided by the insurance are available upon reasonable request by the head of the department Prof. Dr. Albert Nienhaus (a.nienhaus@uke.de).

Authors' contributions
CW and AN developed the study design. DW and CW conducted the data collection, CW and AN conducted the data analysis. The interpretation of the data was made by DW, CW and AN. CW wrote the manuscript, with significant contribution from the other authors. Uncertainties were discussed between the authors regularly. AN revised the manuscript critically for important intellectual content and gave final approval for the version to be published. All authors read and approved the final manuscript and gave approval for publication.

Ethics approval and consent to participate
The study was not submitted to an ethic commission as only anonym routine data of an insurance were used and no personal data were collected and no medical test was performed in the scope of the study. In accordance with the Professional Code for Physicians in Hamburg (Art. 15, 1., Status of 10.03.2014) and the Chamber Legislation for Medical Professions in the Federal State of Hamburg (HmbKGH) it is only necessary to obtain advice on questions of professional ethics and professional conduct from an Ethics Committee if data which can be traced to a particular individual is being used in a research project. However, the study was approved by the data protection board of the insurance which provided the data.

Competing interests
The authors declare that they have no competing interests.

Publisher's Note

Publikation 3

Westermann *et al. Journal of Occupational Medicine and Toxicology* (2018) 13:16

Page 8 of 8

Author details
[1]Competence Centre for Epidemiology and Health Services Research for Healthcare Professionals (CVcare), Institute for Health Services Research in Dermatology and Nursing (IVDP), University Medical Centre Hamburg-Eppendorf (UKE), Martinistr. 52, 20146 Hamburg, Germany. [2]Department of Occupational Medicine, Hazardous Substances and Public Health, Institution for Statutory Accident Insurance and Prevention in the Health and Welfare Services (BGW), Pappelallee 33-37, 22089 Hamburg, Germany.

Received: 8 January 2018 Accepted: 8 May 2018
Published online: 25 May 2018

References
1. Askarian M, Yadollahi M, Kuochak F, Danaei M, Vakili V, Momeni M. Precautions for health care workers to avoid hepatitis B and C virus infection. The international journal of occupational and environmental medicine. 2011;2(4):191–8.
2. Global Hepatitis Report 2017. Geneva: World Health Organization; 2017. Licence: CC BY-NC-SA 3.0 IGO. http://www.who.int/hepatitis/publications/global-hepatitis-report2017/en/. Accessed 15 Sept 2017.
3. Sarrazin C, Berg T, Buggisch P, Dollinger MM, Hinrichsen H, Hofer DH, et al. Aktuelle Empfehlung zur Therapie der chronischen Hepatitis C S3 guideline hepatitis C addendum. Z Gastroenterol. 2015;53:320–34.
4. Ingilz P, Christensen S, Kimhofer T, Hueppe D, Lutz T, Schewe K, Busch H, Schmutz G, Wehmeyer MH, Boesecke C, et al. Sofosbuvir and Ledipasvir for 8 weeks for the treatment of chronic hepatitis C virus (HCV) infection in HCV-Monoinfected and HIV-HCV-Coinfected individuals: results from the German hepatitis C cohort (GECCO-01). Clinical infectious diseases: an official publication of the Infectious Diseases Society of America. 2016; 63(10):1320–4.
5. Lubel J, Strasser S, Stuart KA, Dore G, Thompson A, Pianko S et al. Real-world efficacy and safety of ritonavir-boosted paritaprevir, ombitasvir, dasabuvir +/– ribavirin for hepatitis C genotype 1 - final results of the REV1TAL study. Antivir Ther. 2017;22(8):699–710. https://doi.org/10.3851/IMP3168.
6. Sarrazin C, Berg T, Ross RS, Schirmacher P, Wedemeyer H, Neumann U, et al. Prophylaxis, diagnosis and therapy of hepatitis C virus (HCV) infection: the German guidelines on the management of HCV infection. Zeitschrift fur Gastroenterologie. 2010;48(2):289–351.
7. Westbrook RH, Dusheiko G. Natural history of hepatitis C. J Hepatol. 2014; 61(1 Suppl):S58–68.
8. Gonzalez-Grande R, Jimenez-Perez M, Gonzalez Arjona C, Mostazo TJ. New approaches in the treatment of hepatitis C. World Journal of Gastroenterology : WJG. 2016;22(4):1421–32.
9. Tada T, Kumada T, Toyoda H, Kiriyama S, Tanikawa M, Hisanaga Y et al. Viral eradication reduces all-cause mortality in patients with chronic hepatitis C virus infection: a propensity score analysis. Liver Int. 2016;36:817–26. https://doi.org/10.1111/liv.13071.
10. Nienhaus A, Kesavachandran C, Wendeler D, Haamann F, Dulon M. Infectious diseases in healthcare workers - an analysis of the standardised data set of a German compensation board. J Occup Med Toxicol. 2012;7(1):8.
11. Dulon ML, Lisiak B, Wendeler D, Nienhaus A, Occupational infectious diseases in healthcare workers. Data from the institution for statutory accident insurance and prevention in the health and welfare services. Zbl Arbeitsmed. 2014;65:210–6.
12. Westermann C, Dulon M, Wendeler D, Nienhaus A. Hepatitis C among healthcare personnel: secondary data analyses of costs and trends for hepatitis C infections with occupational causes. J Occup Med Toxicol. 2016;11:52.
13. Swart E, Bitzer EM, Gothe H, Harling M, Hoffmann F, Horenkamp-Sonntag D et al. [A Consensus German Reporting Standard for Secondary Data Analyses, Version 2 (STROSA-STandardisierte BerichtsROutine fur SekundardatenAnalysen)]. Gesundheitswesen (Bundesverband der Ärzte des Öffentlichen Gesundheitsdienstes (Germany)). 2016.
14. Cohen J, Cohen P, West SG, Aiken LS. Applied multiple regression/correlation analysis for the behavioral sciences (3rd ed.). Mahwah: Lawrence Erlbaum; 2003.
15. Nuno Solinis R, Arratibel Ugarte P, Rojo A, Sanchez GY. Value of treating all stages of chronic hepatitis C: a comprehensive review of clinical and economic evidence. Infectious diseases and therapy. 2016;5(4):491–508.
16. Stahmeyer JT, Krauth C, Bert F, Pfeiffer-Vornkahl H, Alshuth U, Huppe D, et al. Costs and outcomes of treating chronic hepatitis C patients in routine care - results from a nationwide multicenter trial. J Viral Hepat. 2016;23(2): 105–15.
17. Backus LI, Belperio PS, Shahoumian TA, Loomis TP, Mole LA. Comparative effectiveness of ledipasvir/sofosbuvir +/– ribavirin vs. ombitasvir/paritaprevir/ritonavir + dasabuvir +/– ribavirin in 6961 genotype 1 patients treated in routine medical practice. Aliment Pharmacol Ther. 2016;44(4):400–10.
18. Lawitz E, Makara M, Akarca US, Thuluvath PJ, Preotescu LL, Varunok P, et al. Efficacy and safety of Ombitasvir, Paritaprevir, and ritonavir in an open-label study of patients with genotype 1b chronic hepatitis C virus infection with and without cirrhosis. Gastroenterology. 2015;149(4):971–80.e1.
19. Zeuzem S. Treatment options in hepatitis C. Dtsch Arztebl Int. 2017; 114(1–02):11–21.
20. Zimmermann R, Kollan C, Ingiliz P, Mauss S, Schmidt D, Bremer V. Real-world treatment for chronic hepatitis C infection in Germany: analyses from drug prescription data, 2010–2015. J Hepatol. 2017;67(1):15–22.
21. Schäfer M, Schwaiger M. Incidence, Pathoetiology and treatment of interferon-α induced neuro-psychiatric side Effetcs. Fortschr Neurol Psychiatr. 2003;71(09):469–76.
22. Slim J, Afridi MS. Managing adverse effects of interferon-alfa and ribavirin in combination therapy for HCV. Infect Dis Clin N Am. 2012;26(4):917–29.
23. 14th Congress for Hospital Hygiene 2018, Berlin, March 18–21, 2018. Lecture on March 19 at 2.45 p.m.: [Vision 'zero infections' - can this be achieved in view of the temporal trend in occupational infections? A contribution to the discussion from the perspective of BGW - A. Nienhaus (Hamburg)]. https://www.congress-compact.de/pdf/2018_03_18-21_DGKH_Jahreskongress_Hauptprogramm.pdf. Accessed 10 Apr 2018.
24. Ltd. LHP. THE ECO-HEP REPORT. A macroeconomic overview of viral hepatitis C in Germany https://www.leberhilfe-projekt.de/das-eco-hep-modell.html: Leberhilfe Projekt gUG (Liver Help Project Ltd.); Babette Herder and Achim Kautz; [2.8.2017]. Accssed 15 Sept 2017.
25. Warpakowski A. Hepatitis C: Elimination in Europa möglich. Dtsch Ärztebl International.113(21):-20-.
26. WHO. GLOBAL HEALTH SECTOR STRATEGY ON VIRAL HEPATITIS 2016–2021 [updated 2.8.2017; cited Juni 2016]. Available from: http://www.who.int/hepatitis/strategy2016-2021/ghss-hep/en/. Accessed 17 May 2018.
27. Webster DP, Klenerman P, Dusheiko GM. Hepatitis C. Lancet 2015;385(9973): 1124–1135.

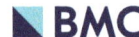

3 Abkürzungsverzeichnis

ArbMedVV	Arbeitsmedizinische Vorsorgeverordnung
AWMF	Arbeitsgemeinschaft Wissenschaftlich Medizinischer Fachgesellschaften
BGW	Berufsgenossenschaft für Gesundheitsdienst und Wohlfahrtspflege
BiG	Beschäftigte im Gesundheitswesen
BioStoffV	Biostoffverordnung
BK	Berufskrankheit
BK-DOK	Berufskrankheiten-Dokumentations-Datenbank
BKV	Berufskrankheiten-Verordnung
BSG	Bundessozialgericht
CHC	Chronische Hepatitis C
DAA	Direct–acting Antiviral Agents
DCV	Daclatasvir
DSV	Dasabuvir
EML	Essential Medicines List
ETR	End of Treatment Response
GECCO	German Hepatitis Cohort
HBV	Hepatitis-B-Virus
HCV	Hepatitis-C-Virus
HIV	Humanes Immundefizienz-Virus
IfSG	Infektionsschutzgesetz
IVD	injizierende (intravenös) Drogenkonsumierende
LDV	Ledipasvir
MdE	Minderung der Erwerbsfähigkeit
MSM	Männer, die Sex mit Männern haben
NS	Nicht strukturell
NSV	Nadelstichverletzung
OBV	Ombitasvir
OPrD	Ombitasvir/Paritaprevir/Ritonavir/Dasabuvir
OR	Odds Ratio
PEG-IFN	Pegyliertes Interferon
PTV	Paritaprevir
UV	Unfallversicherung
RBV	Ribavirin
RNA	Ribonukleinsäure
RTV	Ritonavir
SGB	Sozialgesetzbuch
SMV	Simeprevir
SOF	Sofosbuvir
SVR	Sustained Virological Response
SVR12	Sustained Virological Response zwölf Wochen nach Therapieende
TBC	Tuberkulose
TVR	Telaprevir
WHO	World Health Organization

4 Abbildungsverzeichnis

5 Tabellenverzeichnis